GLOBAL HEALTH

EDITED BY
BRIAN D. NICHOLSON
JUDY MCKIMM
ANN K. ALLEN

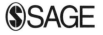

Los Angeles | London | New Delhi
Singapore | Washington DC

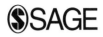

Los Angeles | London | New Delhi
Singapore | Washington DC

SAGE Publications Ltd
1 Oliver's Yard
55 City Road
London EC1Y 1SP

SAGE Publications Inc.
2455 Teller Road
Thousand Oaks, California 91320

SAGE Publications India Pvt Ltd
B 1/I 1 Mohan Cooperative Industrial Area
Mathura Road
New Delhi 110 044

SAGE Publications Asia-Pacific Pte Ltd
3 Church Street
#10-04 Samsung Hub
Singapore 049483

Editor: Alex Clabburn
Associate Editor: Emma Milman
Production editor: Katie Forsythe
Copyeditor: Michelle Clark
Proofreader: Thea Watson
Indexer: Elske Janssen
Marketing manager: Camille Richmond
Cover design: Wendy Scott
Typeset by: C&M Digitals (P) Ltd, Chennai, India
Printed and bound by CPI Group (UK) Ltd,
Croydon, CR0 4YY

Library of Congress Control Number: 2015938117

British Library Cataloguing in Publication data

A catalogue record for this book is available from the British Library

ISBN 978-1-4462-8249-6
ISBN 978-1-4462-8250-2 (pbk)

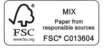

WITHDRAWN

GLOBAL HEALTH

SAGE was founded in 1965 by Sara Miller McCune to support the dissemination of usable knowledge by publishing innovative and high-quality research and teaching content. Today, we publish over 900 journals, including those of more than 400 learned societies, more than 800 new books per year, and a growing range of library products including archives, data, case studies, reports, and video. SAGE remains majority-owned by our founder, and after Sara's lifetime will become owned by a charitable trust that secures our continued independence.

Los Angeles | London | New Delhi | Singapore | Washington DC

CONTENTS

ABOUT THE EDITORS

Brian D. Nicholson is a GP and Clinical Fellow based at the Nuffield Department for Primary Care Health Sciences at the University of Oxford. He intercalated in International Health as a medical student and worked as a research assistant to Professor John Walley at the Nuffield Centre for International Health and Development. He co-founded almamata.org.uk, a not-for-profit network providing information on training, careers, education and research in global health. His current research focuses on the optimization of systems for cancer diagnosis and understanding differences in cancer outcomes between countries. He has received funding from the National Institute for Health Research and Cancer Research UK. Brian sees cancer control in low- to middle-income countries as a one of the major global health challenges ahead.

Judy McKimm is Director of Strategic Educational Development and Professor of Medical Education at Swansea University, working internationally in health professions education. From 2011–2014, she was Dean of Medical Education at Swansea and, from 2007–2011, worked in New Zealand at the University of Auckland and as Pro-Dean, Health and Social Care, at the Unitec Institute of Technology. She trained as a nurse and worked in medical education from 1994–2004, latterly as Director of Undergraduate Medicine at Imperial College, London, leading the development and implementation of a new undergraduate medical programme. From 2004–2005, as Higher Education Academy Senior Adviser, she was responsible for developing and implementing the accreditation of professional development programmes for teachers in higher education. She has worked on over 60 international health workforce and education reform projects in Central Asia, Portugal, Greece, Bosnia and Herzegovina, Macedonia, Australia, the Pacific and the Middle East. She publishes widely on medical education and leadership.

Ann K. Allen retired from her post as Senior Lecturer at the Institute of Medical Education, Cardiff University, in 2013. Previously she was Director of Cardiff University's Master of Public Health Programme. She holds postgraduate degrees in sociology, anthropology, education and development management and has worked in many developing countries as a consultant for project evaluation, health promotion and curriculum design. Her book *Research Skills for Medical Students* was published by Sage in 2012. As a consultant with the Open University, she worked with Ethiopian academics from 2013 until 2014 to develop the curriculum and learning materials for a Master of Human Resources for Health course. She continues to contribute (as a member of the leadership group and an online tutor) to the online People's Open Access Education Initiative (Peoples-uni), which aims to offer high-quality and low-cost education in public health to assist with public health capacity-building.

ABOUT THE CONTRIBUTORS

Stephen Allen

Professor of Paediatrics, Liverpool School of Tropical Medicine, Liverpool, UK, and International Officer, Royal College of Paediatrics and Child Health, London, UK.

Stefi Barna

Lecturer in Global Health, Norwich Medical School, University of East Anglia, UK.

Philippa K. Bird

Principal Research Fellow, Bradford Institute for Health Research, UK.

Colin S. Brown

Academic Clinical Fellow in Infectious Diseases, Centre of Clinical Infection and Diagnostics Research, Department of Infectious Diseases and Infectious Diseases Lead for the King's Sierra Leone Partnership, King's Centre for Global Health, King's College London, UK.

Philip Cotton

Principal, College of Medicine and Health Sciences, University of Rwanda, Rwanda, Africa.

Subodh Dave

Associate Dean, Royal College of Psychiatrists, and Honorary Associate Professor, University of Nottingham, and Consultant Psychiatrist, Derby, UK.

Nisha Dogra

Professor of Psychiatry Education and Honorary Consultant in Child and Adolescent Psychiatry, Greenwood Institute of Child Health, University of Leicester, UK.

Alison Fiander

Professor and Honorary Chair in Obstetrics and Gynaecology, School of Medicine, Cardiff University, UK, and Clinical Lead for Leading Safe Choices, a RCOG initiative to improve global women's health.

Trevor Gibbs

Independent Professor of Medical Education and Primary Care and WHO Consultant in Medical Education, Adolescent Health and Primary Care.

Anu Goenka

Registrar in Paediatrics, Royal Manchester Children's Hospital, UK.

Jason Horsley

Consultant in Public Health, Sheffield City Council, and Honorary Senior Lecturer in Public Health, University of Sheffield, Sheffield, UK.

Rachel Jenkins

Emeritus Professor of Epidemiology and International Mental Health Policy, Institute of Psychiatry, King's College London, UK.

Ann John

Clinical Associate Professor, Swansea University Medical School, Wales, UK and Honorary Consultant in Public Health, Public Health Wales.

Chris Lavy

Professor of Orthopaedic and Tropical Surgery, Nuffield Department of Orthopaedics, Rheumatology and Musculoskeletal Sciences (NDORMS), University of Oxford, UK.

Dan Magnus

Paediatrician, Bristol Children's Hospital, Bristol, UK.

David Mant

Emeritus Professor of General Practice, Nuffield Department of Primary Care Health Sciences, University of Oxford, UK.

Michelle McLean

Professor and Associate Dean of External Engagement and International Marketing, Faculty of Health Sciences and Medicine, Bond University, Queensland, Australia.

Tolib Mirzoev

Associate Professor of International Health Policy and Systems, Nuffield Centre for International Health and Development, University of Leeds, UK.

Nyengo Mkandawire

Professor of Orthopaedics and Head of Surgery, College of Medicine, University of Malawi, Blantyre, Malawi, Africa.

Rosemary Morgan

Research Fellow, Johns Hopkins Bloomberg School of Public Health, Baltimore, Maryland, USA.

Godfrey Muguti

Professorial Chair, Department of Surgery, College of Health Sciences, University of Zimbabwe, Africa.

Rob Mitchell

Emergency Medicine Registrar, Royal Brisbane and Women's Hospital, Australia. Associate Lecturer, School of Medicine, University of Queensland, Australia.

Amy Neilson

Medical Doctor, Médecins Sans Frontières, Health Delegate, Australian Red Cross, and General Practitioner and Locum Senior Medical Officer (Emergency Medicine), Australia.

William Newsholme

Consultant in Infectious Diseases, General Medicine and Infection Control, Guy's and St Thomas' Hospital, London, UK. Honorary Senior Lecturer, King's Centre for Global Health, King's College London, UK.

Georgina Phillips

Emergency Physician, Coordinator of International Programmes, St Vincent's Hospital, Melbourne, Australia, and Honorary Lecturer, University of Melbourne, Australia.

Kate E. Pickett

Professor of Inequalities in Health, Department of Health Sciences, University of York, UK.

Sarah Walpole

NIHR Academic Clinical Fellow in Medical Education at Hull York Medical School and Cardiology Specialist Registrar at Hull Hospitals.

Dileep Wijeratne

Senior Registrar in Obstetrics and Gynaecology Registrar, Bradford Royal Infirmary, Yorkshire, UK, and former Resident Obstetrician and Gynaecologist, Bawku Hospital, Northern Ghana, Africa.

Merlin Willcox

Clinical Researcher, Nuffield Department of Primary Care Health Sciences, University of Oxford, UK.

Bhanu Williams

Consultant Paediatrician, London North West Healthcare NHS Trust, Harrow, UK.

Rhys Williams

Emeritus Professor of Clinical Epidemiology, Swansea University Medical School, Wales, UK.

Andrea Williamson

Senior Clinical University Teacher, University of Glasgow, Scotland, UK.

LIST OF ACRONYMS

ADHD	attention deficit hyperactivity disorder
AFEM	African Federation for Emergency Medicine
AMR	antimicrobial resistance
ART	antiretroviral therapy
CD4	cluster of differentiation 4 – a glycoprotein found on the surface of immune cells
CHD	coronary heart disease
CHE	complex humanitarian emergencies
CHN	community health nurse
CHPS	community-based health and planning services
CHWs	community health workers
CO_2	carbon dioxide
COPD	chronic obstructive pulmonary disease
COSECSA	College of Surgeons of East Central and Southern Africa
CSOs	civil society organizations
D&C	dilatation and curettage
DAH	development assistance for health
DALYs	disability-adjusted life years
DFID	Department for International Development
DOT-HAART	directly observed therapy with highly active antiretroviral therapy
DOTS	directly observed treatment, short-course
DSM	*Diagnostic and Statistical Manual of Mental Disorders*
EC	emergency care
ECDC	European Centre for Disease Prevention and Control
ELRHA	Enhancing Learning and Research for Humanitarian Assistance
EM	emergency medicine

EOC	essential obstetric care
EPI	Expanded Programme on Immunization
ETAT	Emergency Triage Assessment and Treatment
FBOs	faith-based organizations
FMTs	foreign medical teams
GBD	Global Burden of Disease
GDP	gross domestic product
GEC	global emergency care
GECC	Global Emergency Care Collaborative
GHWA	Global Health Workforce Alliance
GOBI FFF	growth monitoring, oral rehydration, breastfeeding, immunization, family spacing, food supplements and female education
HAI	hospital-acquired infection
HCAI	healthcare-associated infection
HIC	high-income countries
HIV/AIDS	human immunodeficiency virus and acquired immune deficiency syndrome
HMIS	health management information systems
HRH	human resources for health
IASC	Inter-Agency Standing Committee
ICD	*International Classification of Diseases*
ICRC	International Committee of the Red Cross
ICU	intensive care unit
IEM	international emergency medicine
IFEM	International Federation for Emergency Medicine
IFMSA	International Federation of Medical Students' Associations
IFRC	International Federation of Red Cross and Red Crescent Societies
IMCI	Integrated Management of Childhood Illness
INGOs	international non-governmental organizations
IPCC	Intergovernmental Panel on Climate Change
IPT	intermittent preventive therapy
IT	information technology
ITNs	insecticide-treated bed nets
JFS	Joint Funding Scheme

KEHPCA	Kenya Hospices and Palliative Care Association
LICs	low-income countries
LMICs	low- and middle-income countries
LTCs	long-term conditions
MCH	maternal and child health
MDGs	Millennium Development Goals
MDR	multi-drug resistant
MDR-TB	multi-drug resistant tuberculosis
MERS-CoV	Middle East respiratory syndrome coronavirus
MMR	maternal mortality ratio
MOHSW	Ministry of Health and Social Welfare (Tanzania, Ethiopia)
MRSA	meticillin-resistant *Staphylococcus aureus*
MSF	Médecins Sans Frontières
NCDs	non-communicable diseases
NDM1	New Delhi metallo-beta-lactamase-1
NGO	non-governmental organization
NHS	National Health Service
NSPCC	National Society for the Prevention of Cruelty to Children
NTDs	neglected tropical diseases
OCHA	Office for the Coordination of Humanitarian Affairs
PCV	pneumococcal conjugate vaccines
PEPFAR	President's Emergency Plan for AIDS Relief (USA)
PHC	primary healthcare
PLWHA	people living with HIV or AIDS
PM	project management
PMTCT	prevention of mother-to-child transmission
PPE	personal protective equipment
ProMED	Programme for Monitoring Emerging Diseases
RAS	refused asylum seekers
RDTs	rapid diagnostic tests
SAM	severe acute malnutrition
SAP	sustainable action planning
SARS	severe acute respiratory syndrome

SDGs	Sustainable Development Goals
SSCL	surgical safety checklist
START	strategic timing of antiretroviral treatment
STAR CHPS	Supportive Technical Assistance for Revitalizing Community-based Health Planning and Services
SWAps	Sector Wide Approaches
TB	tuberculosis
TBAs	traditional birth attendants
TDR-TB	totally drug resistant tuberculosis
TRPCCC	Trent Region Palliative and Continuing Care Centre
UASC	unaccompanied asylum-seeking child
UFM	under-five mortality
UHC	universal health coverage
UK	United Kingdom
UN	United Nations
UNDP	United Nations Development Programme
UNFPA	United Nations Population Fund
UNICEF	United Nations Children's Fund
USAID	United States Agency for International Development
VRE	vancomycin-resistant *Enterococcus*
VSO	Voluntary Service Overseas
WACS	West African College of Surgeons
WHO	World Health Organization
WHO-AIMS	World Health Organization Assessment Instrument for Mental Health Systems
WISN	workload indicators of staffing need
XDR-TB	extensively drug resistant tuberculosis
YLDs	years lived with disabilities
YLLs	years of life lost

FOREWORD

It is appropriate that the publication of this excellent book should coincide with the launch of the United Nations' Sustainable Development Goals (SDGs). The UN has hailed its predecessor, the Millennium Development Goals (MDGs) 'the most successful anti-poverty movement in history'. Some might not agree entirely but the MDGs have undoubtedly had a significant impact in reducing extreme poverty, delivering safe water, improving access to health care and increasing the number of children going to school and much more.

The SDGs take a broader view of global well-being but the challenges for the next 15 years will be even greater and the human resources needed to achieve these goals will challenge us all. In addition a growing global population, persistent conflict and warfare and an increasingly unstable climate will add to the barriers to achieving health equity. I am delighted to see a growing interest in global health among students who have grown up in a much more connected and a smaller world. It is our duty to nurture this interest, guide these students with their careers and ensure that their education and professional development is embedded in a socially accountable approach.

Global health is now firmly on undergraduate curricula, yet much still needs to be done to prepare our students for a more 'local' world where students not only need to understand global health issues but also need to develop cultural competences required to work in a multifaceted environment. While some students will choose to work in low- and middle-income countries, all will live and work in a multicultural and multiethnic society with diverse problems previously alien to past generations of health care workers. The migration of vast numbers of refugees and displaced people across continents has ensured that other people's health issues have now become everyone's.

Some of the greatest challenges will be in the rural and remote areas. We increasingly view the world from an urban-centric perspective, despite that fact that nearly half the world's population is rural and the greatest concentrations of extreme poverty remain at the periphery of health care in isolated communities. It will be these areas, which will offer the biggest challenges to the goal of Universal Health Coverage (UHC). The WONCA (World Organization of Family Doctors) Working Party on Rural Practice has developed a *Rural Medical Education Guidebook*; designed for educators to develop appropriate rurally based undergraduate and postgraduate education aimed at promoting rural practice and rural choices for students and doctors in training. It is also committed to developing global student networks as a way of fostering an understanding of global rural health. I was delighted that the needs of rural and isolated communities are highlighted as a challenge in the text.

I must congratulate the editors and authors for producing a much-needed book, which fills a gap and meets the increasing need for global health educational material. The book provides the ideal introductory text for global health with highlighted key points, contextual references, case studies and guides to further study. I will certainly recommend it to my students as a gateway to global health. The book will also become a resource for postgraduate students and those health care professionals planning to work abroad.

Much success has already been achieved but this book will help consolidate global heath in undergraduate and postgraduate curricula across higher education and professional development.

Dr John Wynn-Jones

Chair WONCA Working Party on Rural Practice

Past President and Founder European Rural and Isolated Practitioners Association

Senior Lecturer in Rural and Global Health, Keele Medical School

INTRODUCTION

BRIAN D. NICHOLSON, JUDY MCKIMM, ANN K. ALLEN

BACKGROUND AND CONTEXT

Most healthcare students and professionals spend some time working or studying overseas, whether it is on an elective, a year out, an exchange or a study visit. International agencies, such as the World Bank, United Nations Development Programme (UNDP), as well as international non-governmental organizations (INGOs), retain health and population as key development themes that attract graduates from social science and engineering disciplines. For universities and the students who study in them, social accountability is becoming more important, not only at the level of governance and community engagement but also for individuals who are developing their professional identities (Woollard and Boelen, 2012). An understanding of global health issues and health management is therefore essential. It is equally vital that students and professionals understand the impact of global health on medicine and healthcare in the UK and other countries.

Globalization and technological developments are changing both professional and social practices in ways that require graduates to be able to live and work in settings that are culturally diverse and subject to environmental and disease threats arising from industrial and urban growth that can only be managed through international collaboration. Demographic change (the ageing, growth and urbanization of populations) is taking place in circumstances that are resource-constrained. The importance of empowering both individuals and communities to improve conditions that impact health is increasingly recognized. Many health professionals work and travel in countries outside those in which they were born or trained and, with increasing international travel and migration patterns, health issues that were once seen only in certain countries are now encountered by health professionals around the world.

We live and work in a 'global village', so students and health professionals need to be aware of the health issues that people around the world face because of poverty, inequalities, climate change, famine, conflict, migration patterns and demographic shifts. They need also to understand how policy decisions relating to trade, land use and energy interact with these to compound deprivation further. Understanding and engaging with global health concerns thus form part of the social accountability, diversity and inclusivity agendas of health and health education organizations worldwide.

GLOBAL HEALTH IS HIGH ON THE AGENDA

In professional standards' frameworks (such as UK General Medical Council, 2009; UK Nursing and Midwifery Council, 2010; UK Public Health Skills and Knowledge Framework, 2014) around the world, graduates are required to demonstrate understanding of and adherence to strategies for addressing global and wider public health issues, including those of indigenous peoples. The presence of global health at the top of the political agenda for high-income countries (such as Crisp, 2007), supported by a stream of documents and resources from the World Health Organization (such as, WHO, 2007; WHO Global Health Observatory www.who.int/gho/en), shows that governments and policymakers recognize moves to address drastic international health and development inequalities are becoming more important for the wider public, too. There is a consequent desire for accessible information about the challenges that really face healthcare provision in low-income countries beyond propaganda and media hysteria, which can obscure important messages, such as those underpinning famine in Africa and swine flu. Health professionals need to understand the perspectives of different countries as they strive to achieve the Millennium Development Goals (MDGs), for example contrasting the 'obesity epidemic' found in many Western countries with extreme poverty, starvation and death through famine and other climate changes in others, understanding differences in access to healthcare or variations in maternal and child health and addressing the chronic disease 'epidemic'.

MDGS AND SUSTAINABLE DEVELOPMENT GOALS

The eight MDGs were produced with the aim of eradicating or alleviating key issues for the world's poorest people by 2015 (see www.un.org/millenniumgoals). They were agreed by all the world's countries and leading development institutions and are to:

1. eradicate extreme poverty and hunger
2. achieve universal primary education
3. promote gender equality and empower women
4. reduce child mortality
5. improve maternal health
6. combat HIV/AIDS, malaria and other diseases
7. ensure environmental sustainability
8. develop a global partnership for development.

In 2015, the United Nations (UN) coordinated efforts to develop Sustainable Development Goals (SDGs) to take forward the work already done around the MDGs. The primary aims are to end poverty, promote prosperity and well-being for all, protect the environment and address climate change (www.un.org/sustainabledevelopment). As well as human health issues, the SDGs consider a much wider range of interrelated aspects, such as establishing safe, dignified and fairly paid jobs, disaster risk reduction, agricultural production, animal diseases and conflict prevention.

HEALTH ISSUES ARE GLOBAL

The concept of global health has moved on from focusing solely on the problems of low- and middle-income countries (LMICs) to encompass health problems with global impact. Problems of non-communicable disease control linked to alcohol, tobacco consumption and obesity, such as cardiovascular diseases and cancer, together with mental health, are joining the more familiar communicable diseases of human immunodeficiency virus (HIV), malaria and tuberculosis (TB) at the top of the research agenda. Environmental issues, too, have expanded beyond concern for the provision of clean water supplies, sanitation and promoting hygiene to include the management of risks associated with trade in food and the misuse of pharmaceuticals, as well as the impact of growing global pollution. Variations in the economic status of individuals and communities with respect to access to mater-nal and child health reflect differences in the social status of women that also may be exacerbated by technological developments, such as ultrasound or IVF. Whether health professionals work internationally or with people from different countries and cultures in their own country, global health issues impact local health care delivery and professional practice daily.

New public–private partnerships, such as the Bill & Melinda Gates Foundation, a growing awareness of climate change and unpredictable politico-economic environments exert new pressures and influence on global health and its governance. Consequently we observe significant shifts in research and development funding worldwide. Diseases that have recently been neglected (such as hookworm, schistoso-miasis, trachoma and leprosy) are moving back up the global agenda and new specialties that require refreshed international collaboration and new expertise appear.

BECOMING AND BEING A GLOBAL PRACTITIONER

Individuals are increasingly urged to be global citizens and health professionals to be 'global practitioners' (McKimm and McLean, 2011). More than ever before, individual health professionals have the means – and, with it, the responsibility – to increase awareness and action through informing colleagues and themselves about global issues, lobbying governments and international actors, forming and support-ing global health pressure groups, volunteering and researching global health puzzles (Frenk et al., 2014).

Health professionals and non-health professionals alike take time out of training to study Masters' and Diploma programmes focused on the challenge of providing equitable healthcare on a global scale. Medical schools have produced hundreds of graduates with additional qualifications in international health, the International Federation of Medical Students' Associations (IFMSA) and Medsin UK have ensured global health is climbing up the agenda on most undergraduate medical curricula and Alma Mata (www.almamata.org.uk) works with the Royal Colleges, lobbies government and informs members on how best to integrate relevant inter-national experience into postgraduate training. There is still, however, much to do to consolidate global health as a core element of undergraduate and postgraduate health professions programmes.

OUR APPROACH

The approach in the book highlights throughout why an understanding of international/global health issues is important and relevant to medicine and healthcare students and trainees, as well as practitioners involved in public health programmes in their own practice in local contexts and those working in other countries and cultures. Although the book discusses global issues, it clearly spells out the links to local practice – indeed, the theme and structure of each chapter is 'local–global–local' (the 'act local, think global' approach).

The book is broken down into three main sections as follows:

Part 1: Providing Care Globally

Chapter 1: Studying and Working in Global Health

Chapter 2: Health Systems

Chapter 3: Human Resources for Health

Part 2: Global Health in Context

Chapter 4: Health Inequalities

Chapter 5: Human Health and the Global Environment

Chapter 6: Climate Change, Long-term Conditions and Sustainable Healthcare

Part 3: Global Health in Practice

Chapter 7: Working with Migrants, Refugees and Asylum Seekers

Chapter 8: Primary Healthcare

Chapter 9: Communicable Diseases

Chapter 10: Non-communicable Diseases, Injuries, Suicide and Self-harm

Chapter 11: Mental Health, Mental Illness and Disability

Chapter 12: Maternal Health

Chapter 13: Child and Adolescent Health

Chapter 14: Global Surgery

Chapter 15: Global Emergency Care and Disaster Health

Chapter 16: Project Planning and Evaluation

CHAPTER STRUCTURE

Each chapter provides a short overview and introduction that sets out the main areas of coverage and context. Case studies are used to illustrate relevant global issues or stories included that refer to both the local and global contexts. 'What is the evidence?' boxes highlight key policy, strategy or clinical innovations and movements. Health promotion and preventive medicine is a theme throughout the book (rather than a separate chapter in its own right) so is woven into each chapter. Issues arising from the management of change and the significance of cultural differences for understanding social behaviour are also common threads. The book introduces relevant theory clearly focused on practical applications in public health and clinical practice. Many acronyms are used in global health so a list of these is given at the beginning of the book.

FINALLY

As we have described, this book provides an introductory text to the challenges and solutions to a range of global health issues for healthcare professionals and practitioners from any discipline (particularly those new to working in international health) wherever they work in the world. We hope that you find it useful and enjoy working in global health as much as we do.

REFERENCES

Crisp, N. (2007) *Global Health Partnerships. The UK Contribution to Health in Developing Countries. Summary and Recommendations*. COI. Available at: www.aspeninstitute. org/sites/default/files/content/images/Global%20Health%20Partnerships%20-%20 Crisp%20Report_0.pdf (accessed 8 October 2015).

Frenk, J., Chen, L., Bhutta, Z.A., Cohen, J., Crisp, N., Evans, T., Fineberg, H., Garcia, P., Ke, Y., Kelley, P., Kistnasamy, B., Meleis, A., Naylor, D., Pablos-Mendez, A., Reddy, S., Scrimshaw, S., Sepulveda, J., Serwadda, D. and Zurayk, H. (2010) 'Health professionals for a new century: transforming education to strengthen health systems in an interdependent world', *The Lancet*, 376(9756): 1923–58.

General Medical Council (2009) *Tomorrow's Doctors*. London: General Medical Council.

McKimm, J. and McLean, M. (2011) 'Developing a global practitioner: Time to act? *Medical Teacher*, 33: 626–631.

Nursing and Midwifery Council (2010) *Standards for Pre-registration Nursing Education*. London: Nursing and Midwifery Council.

Public Health Skills and Knowledge Framework (2014) London: Skills for Health. Available at: www.skillsforhealth.org.uk/resources (accessed 8 October 2015).

Woollard, R. and Boelen, C. (2012) 'Seeking impact of medical schools on health: Meeting the challenges of social accountability', *Medical Education*, 46: 21–27.

World Health Organization (2007) *Everybody's Business: Strengthening Health Systems to Improve Health Outcomes: WHO's Framework for Action*. Geneva: World Health Organization.

PART I
PROVIDING CARE GLOBALLY

1

STUDYING AND WORKING
IN GLOBAL HEALTH

MICHELLE MCLEAN AND TREVOR GIBBS

Chapter overview

After reading this chapter, you will be able to:

- explain why it is important for healthcare students and professionals to be knowledgeable about global health
- describe the qualities and attributes of global healthcare practitioners
- plan an elective overseas
- prepare for working successfully overseas.

INTRODUCTION

Large-scale migration, together with the relative ease of travelling across the globe, improved communication technology, large multinational corporations aggressively recruiting globally and higher education becoming big business, have culminated in an increasing national diversity on all continents. This 'flattening' of our world (that is, globalization) has not only created a mobile healthcare workforce but also led to the notion of *global health*, defined as 'health issues and concerns that transcend national borders, class, race, ethnicity and culture' (Global Health Education Consortium, 2011). While globalization has benefits, our connectedness across continents has also facilitated the spread of disease, with pathogens not recognizing national borders.

Medical and health professions education thus needs to train global health practitioners who can translate their knowledge and experience of global health issues into local action. Not only do graduates need to function as members of multiprofessional teams but they also need to be culturally competent in a world in which peers, patients and colleagues often originate from different parts of the world (McKimm and McLean, 2011).

WHAT PROBLEMS DOES DIVERSITY OF THE PROFESSIONAL WORKFORCE BRING?

Through the use of scenarios informed by our experiences as international educators and the wealth of literature addressing global health, this chapter explores the challenges students and health professionals may face in an ever-flattening world of travel, study and work. Solutions are explored and recommendations made. The chapter also considers the attributes, qualities and skills for working effectively with a wide range of patients and communities in different parts of the world. The scenarios aim to stimulate discussion on the ethics of international engagement and service learning in global health, highlighting issues arising within multidisciplinary and multicultural teams.

STUDENTS: GLOBAL HEALTH ELECTIVES AND INTERNATIONAL HEALTH EXPERIENCES

Possibly the feeling of enhanced connectedness on a global scale and a sense of global community leads students and graduates to seek educational experiences in other cultures to enrich their understanding of healthcare. International electives and exchange opportunities are probably the main vehicle for engaging students in global health.

TYPES OF GLOBAL HEALTH EXPERIENCES

Volunteer work was once the most common international health experience for students. Nowadays, a compulsory healthcare elective (in which students have some choice in where they go) is becoming the norm, partly driven by the need to include global health in the core curriculum and in terms of social accountability. The following are three common types of global health experience.

- **Voluntary** If there is no requirement in the curriculum to undertake an elective, students may choose to volunteer with a range of organizations that work in strife-torn and/or under-resourced areas. Volunteering is often driven by the altruistic motive 'to help those less fortunate'.
- **Compulsory, student-organized** Some universities require students to undertake a compulsory elective, but expect them to arrange this themselves. The downside of such an arrangement is that supervision cannot always be guaranteed, nor can the outcomes for the student or the host community. Often the experience will not be formally assessed.
- **Compulsory, institution-organized** The training institution takes responsibility for students' experiences before, during and after the elective. A memorandum of understanding between the institution and one or more sites in the host country and community ensures reciprocity in terms of an exchange programme for students and academics and the infrastructure for teaching. It also guarantees an appropriate standard of clinical supervision and learning outcomes for students as well as protecting patients. Examples would include the arrangement between the universities of St Andrews (Scotland) and Malawi and Swansea University (Wales) and The Gambia.

Activity 1.1

Read the following scenario about undertaking an elective in a developing country. Make notes of the issues that you think would be important if you were undertaking the elective.

Mary (fourth-year medical student) and Simon (final-year nursing student) have spent the last year planning their elective. They are looking forward to spending three weeks in Uganda, hoping to learn more about healthcare there. Once details of their placement (for example, accommodation, what they would be doing, what to expect, who would supervise them) were agreed with the responsible faculty member at their home institution, it was time to attend to their pre-travel medical issues. They required some vaccinations (yellow fever, hepatitis A) and were provided with anti-malarial prophylaxis and anti-diarrhoeal medication. The British High Commission facilitated the issue of their visas and the British Council in Kampala was informed of the dates of their impending visit and had assured them that there was no political unrest in the country and an election was not due for at least a year.

After a long flight, Mary and Simon were met at the airport and escorted to their some-what basic accommodation adjacent to the district hospital where they would be working. Despite attending orientation sessions before their departure, they were taken aback by local conditions – long queues of extremely ill patients, many of whom were children who had waited all day; a poorly stocked pharmacy; worn linen; and an obvious shortage of health-care professionals. Also, although a local paediatrician and the Matron of the hospital had been assigned as their supervisors, the doctor was called away urgently to sort out a family crisis at the end of their first week. So, as there was no other paediatrician and the Matron was too busy, Mary and Simon had to work with the nursing staff, many of whom did not speak English and were often called to assist elsewhere. Occasionally, both Mary and Simon were asked to undertake procedures they had not performed previously. As they were told during their pre-departure briefing that they were to work within their scope of practice and level of competence, they often declined. They found it difficult to refuse as there was clearly a need for more help, but they were careful about what they undertook. During two emergency situations, they had to assist a doctor with unfa-miliar surgical procedures as there was no one else. Simon had to act as the senior theatre nurse.

One aspect they both found difficult was obtaining consent for simple procedures, such as taking blood and suturing, as most patients did not speak English. With a shortage of nurses who could translate, they found that they were not always able to obtain patient consent, but decided that they were doing no harm and their involvement was beneficial to patients' health outcomes.

Comment

Despite Mary and Simon planning their elective thoroughly, their plans went somewhat awry. They were in a poorly resourced district hospital with no supervisor and a shortage of health professionals. Although they were acutely aware of their scope of practice and competence, they did assist with some unfamiliar operations and carried out a small number of procedures that they felt they were not competent to perform. Patient consent and talking to patients were difficult because of the language barrier, but they believed that they were causing no harm to the patients. Their elective appeared to be uneventful in terms of personal health and safety issues. Mary's decision to pair up with Simon during the elective was wise.

PLANNING AND UNDERTAKING THE ELECTIVE

Whatever your healthcare and professional background, thorough planning is critical to ensure that you are adequately prepared personally and professionally (Lumb and Murdoch-Eaton, 2014).

- Make sure that you know the country well, particularly the location in which you will be working, including its climate. Check the country's political stability via the Foreign Office website or equivalent. Ethnic violence is not uncommon in many countries, but may not always be in the news.
- Anticipate the unexpected (being robbed, sick, involved in a motor vehicle accident) and plan what you would do. If you know of others who have visited the area, ask their advice.
- Try to link up with a local volunteer organization working in the country, even if you have arranged the elective through your institution.

Outlined below are key issues that you need to reflect on when planning an international elective as a future healthcare professional.

- Reflect on why you have chosen this particular elective and its location. Although altruism is laudable, evaluate whether or not your aspirations are reasonable in terms of your personal development and if there are beneficial outcomes for the hosting facility and community. At the very least, your presence should 'do no harm' and should incur no costs to the hosts.
- In some instances, if you are undertaking volunteer work or a compulsory elective at a facility or in a community not organized by your institution, there may be out-of-pocket costs for the community or facility. As a minimum, you may be expected, implicitly or not, to reimburse your hosts for the professional time and resources used. You may also be expected to bring gifts for your hosts.
- You will need to know in advance what activities you will be undertaking. These should match your level of competence. Working within your scope of practice is important particularly if you are still in the early stages of your studies as you will not be competent to carry out many clinical procedures. If you are required to specify a specialty area in your application, be aware that some disciplines (such as obstetrics and midwifery, emergency medicine, surgery) could result in you being asked to work outside your scope of practice, risking exposure to blood-borne pathogens. There should be a clear understanding between you and your point of contact (an administrator at the facility you will visit, for example), as well as with an academic at your training institution. Working beyond your competence level is a patient safety issue and could lead to unethical practice.
- Before departure, ascertain what resources are available. Speaking to someone who has visited previously gives you a better understanding of what to expect. In a low-resource country, one should always expect patient:health professional ratios to be much higher than in Western countries and there may be equipment and medicine shortages.
- Students should always maintain the same ethical standards they would at home. These include honesty and integrity, treating patients with dignity and respect,

placing their needs above all else and being non-discriminatory and culturally accepting. All healthcare students have a duty to report any unprofessional or unethical behaviour of their peers during electives. Writing down such events helps as, later, you are asked to provide evidence.

- Not only is being able to communicate with patients and healthcare professionals important to developing a working relationship but there are also implications in terms of ethical principles. Wherever you practise, obtaining patient (informed) consent before touching them or undertaking any procedure is paramount. This can be difficult if there is a language difference. Learn some key words and phrases in the local language to help with this. It is sometimes possible to acquire the services of someone to translate, but you need to ensure that they translate authentically rather than telling you what he or she thinks you want to hear. Bear in mind that providing this service is an additional cost for the hosting facility and may not be appropriate if staffing is stretched.

- Familiarize yourself with the local customs and traditions of the country, particularly the region you intend visiting. In many countries, different tribes and ethnic groups exist. Locals might consult a traditional healer and use traditional medicines before seeing a Western-trained doctor. Families may be part of the decision-making process and, in countries where there are distinct gender roles, males may make decisions on behalf of the women in the family. If you are female, this may influence how you are perceived by male patients or family members. In many parts of the world, the doctor still retains power within the healthcare team, with nurses clearly lower in the hierarchy. Certain clinical practices, such as female circumcision, may be part of the culture of the country you intend visiting. Prior to departure, reflect on how you will deal with such an issue.

- Familiarize yourself with the major health risks of the region you plan to visit (such as yellow fever, malaria, schistosomiasis, tuberculosis, sunburn, heatstroke). All forms of hepatitis and HIV are prevalent in many places. Preventing needlestick injuries therefore becomes paramount. Also, plan how you will address lack of access to potable water. Below are some suggestions.

  o Check your government's travel website for which vaccinations are required and ensure that these are done before you leave.
  o If HIV is a risk, take your own supply of latex gloves and use double gloves when dealing with patients. It is advisable to carry post-exposure prophylaxis for HIV in case of a needlestick injury and in case of being raped.
  o Depending on location, you may need to take the appropriate malarial chemoprophylactics and provide your own mosquito net. Make sure that you can tolerate the medication. If in any doubt, seek medical advice *before* you leave. It is also advisable to take your own supply of antibiotics, as well as anti-emetic and anti-diarrhoeal medication.
  o Your travel insurance should cover evacuation in the event of emergency surgery (such as an appendectomy or if you are involved in a motor vehicle accident).

- Be aware of personal safety issues.

  o Never underestimate risks to your personal safety, particularly if you are travelling alone.
  o Check your government's website for the latest 'risks' associated with travel to the country you have chosen.

o   Ensure that your embassy or consulate is aware of your impending visit and has comprehensive details (location, telephone numbers, next of kin and so on). If your country has a consulate or embassy in the country in which you will be working, make contact before and on arrival. Inform the embassy or consulate of your arrival and departure dates.

o   Carry emergency contact details on your person (of someone in the country you are visiting or a family member at home, for example). If possible, have these details translated into the local language.

o   Make sure your mobile phone has international coverage in case of an emergency. Consider phoning parents, relatives or friends on a regular basis.

o   Consider undertaking the elective in pairs. If you are a woman, consider a male companion (as Simon and Mary did). Carry condoms in case of rape. You may not be able to prevent the rape, but you might be able to convince your assailant to wear a condom or allow you to use a female version.

RETURNING FROM YOUR ELECTIVE

As a minimum, on returning from your elective, you should do the following.

- Undertake a full medical if you are experiencing any abnormal symptoms, such as persistent diarrhoea or night sweats. Checking for tuberculosis is paramount.
- Debrief with a faculty member at your institution. This is particularly important if you have witnessed a professional or traumatic event or have perhaps been knowingly or inadvertently engaged in what you might consider unprofessional conduct. You may also have been a victim of or witnessed violence or political unrest.

THE ETHICS OF GLOBAL HEALTH ELECTIVES

Socially accountable education for health professionals should incorporate teaching and learning experiences such as global health electives that allow students to develop the skills required to work as future global citizens. As a minimum, their involvement should 'do no harm' to host communities and should incur no costs for the facilities where they work. Ideally, both parties should benefit from the experience (Evert et al., 2008).

Numerous benefits for students undertaking international electives have been espoused (sometimes without sufficient evidence), such as better understanding of tropical diseases, cultural awareness, health systems and public health, clinical skills, attitudes, personal and professional development (Thompson et al., 2003). Students themselves have reported that they had had no significant impact on the community or were unable to assess the impact of their contact, due, in part, to the short-term nature (a few weeks) of many electives (Stys, Hopman and Carpenter, 2013). As social accountability is being placed in a more prominent position within the mission of schools of medicine and health professions education, all institutions should evaluate the impact of their students moving into the wider global community during electives.

--- **Activity 1.2** ---

Identify a potential ethical concern relating to an overseas placement in a developing country and then discuss with a peer or colleague.

Comment

One of the foremost ethical concerns in terms of students working in developing countries is the vulnerability of patients, many of whom may be educationally and socio-economically disadvantaged (Thompson et al., 2003). In situations where clinical supervision is lacking, students may work outside their scope of practice and level of competence, either voluntarily (by, for example, offering to undertake an unfamiliar procedure) or involuntarily (such as in life and death situations). It is easy to imagine how learning can take place at the expense of patients (*BMJ*, 2008: 337):

> Released from oversight he saw an opportunity effectively to practise on a captive population. He altered a prescription written by a local doctor; he photographed patients undergoing intimate procedures without consent; and he performed an unnecessary lumbar puncture because he fancied 'having a go'.

Source: Anon (2008)

RETHINKING GLOBAL HEALTH ELECTIVES

Global health electives as part of the core health professions curriculum should be properly organized and appropriately supervised to train healthcare professionals to both understand global inequity, in terms of resources and access to healthcare, and be willing to contribute to its alleviation. As experiential learning has a strong affective component, particularly if it involves immersion in a foreign culture, the minimum requirements for global health electives should be 'pre-departure briefing and training, measurable outcomes for students, adequate supervision and debriefing on return' (Lumb and Murdoch-Eaton, 2014). Value-added inclusions to these minimum requirements also could incorporate the utilization of international faculty (including the host institution), patients and communities as resources and co-developers of curriculum material, assessment of the elective and evaluation of the engagement.

The best format for electives is a compulsory experience organized by the institution, ideally incorporating a reciprocal exchange programme, such that outcomes can be controlled and assessed, supervisors are always available and with a bi-directional flow of benefits. In such a structured, reciprocal arrangement, the criticism of electives being too short to benefit local communities may be offset by the continuity of students from the same institution picking up where the last group left off and then reporting on the progress of the intervention or project. For students, their experience would also be a structured mentoring engagement.

HEALTH PROFESSIONALS: WORKING ABROAD

Today's health workforce is globally mobile for several reasons:

- availability of postgraduate studies abroad
- recruitment of international faculty for offshore professional training institutions, often in low- and middle-income countries (LMICs)
- health professionals (including volunteers and consultants) working in areas of need
- reciprocal arrangements between institutions for global health electives, requiring academic staff to be trained, to provide training or perhaps to also supervise.

As a result, many hospitals and universities in both high-income countries and emerging economies now have an international complement of culturally diverse staff. Multidisciplinary and multicultural teams are thus common.

Activity 1.3

List some of the issues that a health professional working abroad might face in an unfamiliar culture.

Comment

We don't know what you have identified, but compare your thoughts with the following of Ali, a young Muslim doctor who has just commenced his residency training in the UK.

CASE STUDIES

Case study 1   Working in a culturally different context

Dr Ali is one month into his junior medical residency at a large London teaching hospital. Having spent all his life in a Muslim country in the Middle East, he undertook his medical studies and completed his internship in his home country. In order to be offered this UK post, he had to satisfy a number of General Medical Council requirements, which he duly did.

It is the second week since Ali's wife, Farah, and young son had returned to his home country. Although they had accompanied him when he started, his wife was not happy being away from her sisters and mother and decided to return home, leaving Ali alone in London.

Dr Ali has enjoyed the job so far, meeting a lot of patients from different cultural backgrounds. He is also getting used to many patients being knowledgeable about their illnesses, the fact that he has to ask women to undress and always having to ask patients for their consent before he carries out any examination or investigation.

Tonight, his first time being on call, Ali is asked to attend to a scantily dressed woman who is obviously very inebriated and heavily pregnant. Dr Ali finds this shocking as this situation is foreign to his culture. She refuses to let Ali examine her, accusing him of being a terrorist.

Although the UK is culturally diverse, it is a Western country, which is very different socially and culturally from the more conservative Middle East where Ali was raised according to Islamic principles. With Islam's strict social regulations in terms of dress code, alcohol and marked gender roles, the inebriated, scantily clad pregnant woman in the scenario would have been challenging socially, psychologically and culturally for Ali. Her verbal abuse/accusation would have been unsettling.

In any society, cultural conservatism in terms of 'foreigners' will exist in a proportion of the population. With some of the recent attacks on Westerners by Islamic fundamentalists (killing a British soldier in broad daylight outside his own barracks; IS beheading journalists), anti-Muslim sentiments should not be unexpected. With Ali's wife returning home with their young son, because she felt socially isolated, Ali is now alone in a culturally foreign country.

It is possible that you may empathize with Ali and his wife, either because you are an international student or perhaps you have witnessed a peer or colleague bearing the brunt of a racial or cultural slur.

The following two case studies elaborate on other issues that may arise when health professionals work abroad. Case study 2 depicts a situation faced by many health professionals working in an under-resourced country with poor healthcare provision (Haiti, in this case), while the third scenario describes a young Chinese cardiologist who trained in the UK and has returned to Hong Kong.

Case study 2   Working in a resource-poor country

Since qualifying as a midwife 15 years ago, Maria has had a sense of social responsibility. She has always wanted to use her skills and experience in a less developed country. Now that her family has left home, she has decided to take a three-month sabbatical in Haiti. Having read all about Haiti after the 2010 earthquake, Maria felt that she would be able to provide assistance to a struggling community.

It was a hot day when Maria arrived at her hospital in Port-au-Prince. After settling in, she was given a tour of the maternity facilities by the Head of Maternity services. What she saw and what she was told was not what she expected.

She learned that most of the women arrive at the hospital in an advanced stage of labour, having had little or no antenatal care. This is because many women have to work until the last minute because they are the breadwinners of an extended family. The recent earthquake, the poor health and social conditions and the HIV/AIDS situation has meant that many pregnant women are either unmarried or widowed. Taking one day away from work for antenatal care translates into no money and no food for the rest of the family. The lack of antenatal care means complications associated with pregnancy and delivery are high, with high infant and maternal mortality rates. With the low number of trained midwives and attendant physicians, many healthcare workers are asked to undertake procedures well beyond their competency levels. Many of the Haiti women do not know whether they are HIV positive so healthcare workers must be constantly vigilant.

Many of the tragedies of childbirth, leading either to death or severe birth trauma of the infant, are put down to 'circumstance' or 'life' and the mother and/or relatives are expected to return to normal life as soon as possible. There is little or no counselling or follow-up care. Maria cries herself to sleep most nights.

Maria is a well-qualified, experienced midwife who brings with her a high level of anticipatory care. Her experience suggests that obstetrics and midwifery has moved on considerably since she was a student and within her own understanding. She expects the rest of the world to follow, although maybe not to the same high level. Her experience abroad conflicts with her own training, her own high standards of clinical care and the respect she has for her profession and the patients for whom she is responsible. She finds it difficult to reconcile 'how cheap life is' in Haiti with her own intrinsic values, of life being precious.

Case study 3   Working in a multiprofessional and multicultural team

Dr Peter Wu is excited to be going back to Hong Kong, where he was born just over 30 years ago. He has lived in the UK for most of his life as his parents emigrated when he was only a few months old. His father is proud of Peter, who has followed him into medicine and only recently qualified as a cardiologist. As part of his training and the need to experience his specialty in another country, he is about to spend a year at his father's old hospital in Hong Kong.

During his training in the UK, Peter developed an appreciation of cardiology as a team specialty. He had learned from his first few days of training that everyone on the team had a role and each team member respected the others. Patient safety was their priority. In his new position in Hong Kong, things work differently and, in Peter's opinion, his team does not function efficiently. Is it because the cardiology team is multicultural, comprised of healthcare professionals from different parts of Asia, the Far East and Europe, or is it because the healthcare system places less emphasis on the multidisciplinarity of the team? Either way, communication in the team is less than professional, with senior doctors often barking orders to their juniors and the nurses on the team. There is often considerable disagreement, too, and delays on the ward and in the operating theatres, putting patients' lives at risk.

The third scenario describes the situation of a UK-trained Chinese health professional who returns to his place of birth to find that the hierarchical relationships between the culturally diverse healthcare professionals interfered with service delivery and compromised patients. Although Peter was born in Hong Kong and is Chinese, he was raised and studied in a Western country. Accustomed to working in an efficient team where communication is key, Peter found himself in a very different work environment, one in which teamwork is not valued. He found that the multicultural and multiprofessional team to which he is assigned is hierarchical, with senior doctors still functioning within the paradigm of 'the doctor is always in charge'. There appears to be little respect for the skills of the different members of the team, many of whom are expatriates. Respectful, effective communication seems non-existent.

Health professionals who choose to study or work in a foreign country are faced with many cultural and social issues such as these. A dual responsibility, however, exists when individuals study or work abroad.

- **Responsibility of the student or the healthcare professional** When choosing to study or work abroad, particularly when the culture is very different, there is an onus on the individual to understand the conditions under which he or she will study or work. First-hand information from someone who has studied or worked there is probably the most important means of getting an idea of what awaits. Searching the Internet for blogs or websites might also yield 'must know' information.

- **Responsibility of the host or the employer** The host institution or facility and/or the employer have a responsibility to provide the new recruit with support and assistance during the settling-in period and at work or study. Providing information (local culture, work circumstances) prior to the new student or appointee's arrival would assist the transition. There should be opportunities to ask questions. A contact person to assist with administration, medical requirements and licensing would also go a long way to assisting the new recruit with settling in to studying or working in a new environment.

Activity 1.4

In the light of what you have gleaned from the case studies provided in this chapter, list activities you would undertake to prepare yourself to study or work abroad.

Comment

Hopefully, most of what you identified is listed in the section below. You have probably also identified additional issues because they are important to you.

RECOMMENDATIONS WHEN STUDYING OR WORKING ABROAD

- Familiarize yourself with the community in which you will study or work. Although the population in Western countries is becoming increasingly ethnically diverse, these countries are still largely Christian. Similarly, if you are taking up employment in Asia or the Middle East, for example, and originate from Europe, the UK or North America, you need to ensure that you are *au fait* with the local culture and religions. If you are religious and your culture is important, ensure that you are able to locate a place of worship in the new country to avoid cultural disorientation. Although written from the perspective of working with indigenous communities, Smith's (2007) recommendations are equally applicable to new social contexts in which students or healthcare professionals choose to work or study (see below).
- Research the country extensively to familiarize yourself not just with the medical problems but also the social issues affecting the country. It is the latter that will frequently have the greatest impact on you, perhaps causing distress.
- If you are travelling alone to a new country where you have no friends or relatives, you could become socially isolated. You may be expected to live in a 'compound' if the institution offers housing as part of the remuneration package. Make sure you understand your employment contact. If you are studying, make sure you understand the rules and regulations. Consider how you can make friends or join a local society.
- Be aware of the professional registration regulations of the country where you intend working. As a health professional, be aware that you might have to

travel to your home country, perhaps on an annual basis, to maintain your professional registration.

- Several authors have identified the concerns and implications of foreign students and health professionals not being aware of the intricacies, nuances and colloquialisms of the language in the new country. This could be interpreted by patients and colleagues as a lack of clinical knowledge and skills. In addition, confusion could lead to potential misunderstandings and risks to patients.
- While professionalism is often considered in the same breath as healthcare, some aspects of professionalism are not perceived in the same way across cultures. An area of professionalism that varies considerably is the doctor–patient relationship. In Western countries, a patient-centred approach is favoured over the more doctor-centred, paternalistic approach dominant in many other cultures. This necessarily involves different perceptions relating to informed consent, patient autonomy and patient confidentiality.

What is the evidence?

Padela and colleagues' (2008) exploratory qualitative study, with Muslim physicians trained outside and now practising in the USA, identified the challenge of working with populations whose lifestyles are at odds with Islamic teachings and end-of-life care, as the following extract shows (Padela et al., 2008: 367):

> Several participants suggested that Islam profoundly influenced their practice of medicine, including the specialty they pursued, the type of patients they feel most comfortable managing, and the types of procedures they perform. Neda noted how Islam may affect specialty choice: 'Muslim (male) doctors, not necessarily me … would not go and do obstetrics or gyn[aecology] because they would not really want to see an exposed patient … Muslim women doctors would not go into urology.' Multiple participants commented on prohibited medical procedures – for example Neda listed 'abortion', '[purely] cosmetic procedures' and 'sex change' in this category. Furthermore, several respondents mentioned clinical situations where ethical dilemmas would arise due to their adherence to Islam, specifically relating to end-of-life care. Muhammad felt that 'some Muslim physicians … feel that if we are taking any part in [the] decision making of ending somebody else's life, that's not right. That would be against the religion.' Basheer said, 'We do not do [that] which would terminate their life quickly. We do not take the patients off the ventilator just because the chance is low for their survival.'

In many ways, the UK healthcare system operates in a less hierarchical way than in many other countries. Multidisciplinary teams are an important element in healthcare delivery. For doctors from more hierarchical systems with more definite role distinctions (that is, dimensions of power relations; Hofstede, 1986), this may be challenging. A lack of understanding of the roles and responsibilities of others in the team could interfere with interprofessional relationships and be interpreted as a lack of respect.

--- Activity 1.5 ---

Based on your reading of this chapter, reflect on the qualities needed to study or work abroad and discuss them with a peer or colleague.

Comment

You probably agreed that study or working in other countries is not for everyone. It is therefore important to recognize whether or not it suits you. For some, the circumstances underpinning the move may be extenuating (that is, financial or personal safety issues). It is important, therefore, to be sensitive to the experiences of foreign peers or colleagues even if you would not choose to go abroad yourself. The attributes and qualities of global healthcare practitioners (including those in training) are discussed in the next section.

QUALITIES AND ATTRIBUTES OF GLOBAL HEALTHCARE PRACTITIONERS

Based on our personal experiences as international medical educators, we believe that certain qualities and attributes are required to study and work abroad. Before contemplating the challenge of working abroad, particularly in a different culture, consideration should be given to whether or not the following descriptions apply to you.

- Having uncompromising ethical standards, placing patients and their care above your personal needs (within reason).
- Being resourceful and innovative in circumstances where shortages may exist, but accepting that one is not able to solve the world's problems. One's contributions should serve the needs of the community or immediate patients.
- Remaining emotionally and mentally resilient, especially in the face of futility.
- Embracing diversity, accepting cultural differences and being open to different perspectives.
- Being willing to recognize one's level of competence and not work beyond it, unless the benefit clearly outweighs the potential harm.
- Being prepared to work in a multicultural and multiprofessional team and acknowledge that roles and responsibilities may change, depending on the circumstance.
- Acknowledging the good work done by others, giving credit when it is due.

CONCLUSION

Just as all graduates are expected to meet certain standards before they are allowed to practice, the same should be expected of all students and healthcare professionals, irrespective of where they practice. There is thus a dual responsibility for any healthcare professional working or student studying abroad. Personally, the individual needs to be professionally and culturally competent to manage the task, while the host institution or employer needs to ensure that the individual is provided with adequate information prior to arrival and then receives orientation, training and support. For students, training establishments have a responsibility to protect the host communities, just as students have to understand the potential power they may have over vulnerable populations. Similarly, employers of health professionals, wherever they are in the world, are responsible for ensuring staff members are culturally competent professionals. This should involve agencies at all levels – governments, regulators, employers. Each has a role to support international doctors in their transition to the new social and cultural context. If we are to tackle health inequities, a concerted global effort is required. Although Crisp's (2007) report relates to the UK's contributions to health in low-resource countries, his message is universal: Developing countries have requested partnerships with hospitals and healthcare schools in developed countries, with reciprocity in terms of mutual learning and exchange. Such collaboration across national borders has numerous benefits such as:

1. Improved population health and welfare.
2. Greater cross-cultural awareness.
3. Educational benefits for students of partner institutions.
4. Financial benefits.
5. Enhanced reputation.
6. More efficient, cost-effective service delivery.
7. Enhanced staff motivation (Kanter 2010).

In Hanson and colleagues' (2011) view, global health electives will do little to address historically and politically rooted global health inequities unless critical consciousness is raised through improved global health curricula and appropriate pedagogical strategies. With one of the long-term benefits of student engagement in international health electives being an increased disposition of these students towards primary healthcare and for working in underserved communities (Stys et al., 2013), we, however, need to capitalize on students' enthusiasm and often genuine desire to improve the quality of life of vulnerable populations through international collaboration between funders, health professions schools and host communities.

USEFUL LINKS AND ORGANIZATIONS

AFMC Global Health Resource Group and CFMS Global Health Programme

www.cfms.org/downloads/Pre-Departure%20Guidelines%20Final.pdf

Association of American Medical Colleges, global health learning opportunities

www.aamc.org/services/ghlo

British Medical Association, toolkit of electives

http://bma.org.uk/developing-your-career/medical-student/medical-electives-ethics-toolkit

Canadian Federation of Medical Students, Preparing Medical Students for Electives in Low-Resource Settings: A Template for National Guidelines for Pre-Departure Training

www.cfms.org/index.php/global-health/projects/pre-departure-training.html

Global Consensus for Social Accountability of Medical Schools

http://healthsocialaccountability.org

Harvard Global Health Institute

http://globalhealth.harvard.edu

MedAct (a charity for health professionals and others working to improve health worldwide)

www.medact.org

Medical Electives by Medics Away

http://medicsaway.co.uk

Médecins Sans Frontières

www.msf.org

Medsin UK (a student network and registered charity tackling global and local health inequalities through education, advocacy and community action)

www.medsin.org

The Electives Network

www.electives.net

THEnet (a network of collaborating medical schools experimenting with instructional and institutional innovation to attract, retain and enhance the productivity of health professionals serving disadvantaged populations, usually in remote and rural areas)

http://thenetcommunity.org

Third World Network

www.twnside.org.sg

Work the World

www.worktheworld.co.uk

REFERENCES

Anon (2008) 'Students whose behaviour causes concern: case history', *British Medical Journal*, 337:a2878.http://dx.doi.org/10.1136/bmj.a2874

Crisp, N. (2007) *Global Health Partnerships. The UK Contribution to Health in Developing Countries. Summary and Recommendations*. COI. Available at: www.aspeninstitute.org/sites/default/files/content/images/Global%20Health%20Partnerships%20-%20Crisp%20Report_0.pdf (accessed 8 October 2015).

Evert, J., Stewart, C., Chan, K., Rosenberg, M., Hall, T. et al. (2008) *Developing Residency Training in Global Health: A Guidebook*. San Francisco: Global Health Education Consortium.

Global Health Education Consortium (GHEC) (2011) Available at: http://globalhealtheducation.org/SitePages/Home.aspx (accessed 8 October 2015).

Hanson, L., Harms, S. and Plamondon, K. (2011) 'Undergraduate international medical electives: some ethical and pedagogical considerations', *Journal of Studies in International Education*, 15(2): 171–185.

Hofstede, G. (1986) 'Cultural differences in teaching and learning', *International Journal of Intercultural Relations*, 10(3): 301–320.

Kanter, S.L. (2010) 'International collaborations between medical schools: what are the benefits and risks?' *Academic Medicine,* 85(10): 1547–2548.

Lumb, A. and Murdoch-Eaton, D. (2014) 'Electives in undergraduate medical education: AMEE Guide No. 88', *Medical Teacher,* 36: 557–572.

McKimm, J. and McLean, M. (2011) 'Developing a global health practitioner: time to act?', *Medical Teacher,* 33: 626–631.

Padela, A.I., Shanawani, H., Greenlaw, J., Hamid, H., Aktas, M. and Chin, N. (2008) 'The perceived role of Islam in immigrant Muslim medical practice in the USA: an exploratory qualitative study', *Journal of Medical Ethics,* 34(5): 365–369.

Smith, J.D. (2007) *Australia's Rural and Remote Health: A Social Justice Perspective.* Sydney: Pearson Education. pp. 69–71.

Stys, D., Hopman, W. and Carpenter, J. (2013) 'What is the value of global health electives during medical school?', *Medical Teacher,* 35: 209–218.

Thompson, M., Huntington, M., Hunt, D., Pinsky, L., and Brodie, J. (2003) 'Educational effects of international health electives on U.S. and Canadian medical students and residents: a literature review', *Academic Medicine,* 78(3): 342–347.

HEALTH SYSTEMS

TOLIB MIRZOEV AND ROSEMARY MORGAN

> ### Chapter overview
>
> After reading this chapter you will be able to:
>
> - explain how the definition of health used affects what is included in a health system
> - describe the history of health system development
> - describe how health systems differ
> - evaluate the roles of different actors
> - explain how equity and quality in healthcare delivery can be assured.

INTRODUCTION

How a health system is designed, its resources and mode of delivery ultimately affect population health. Understanding health systems and improving their effectiveness and efficiency often improves health outcomes (Skolnik, 2008), which is particularly relevant within resource-poor settings.

This chapter introduces you to the principles of a systems approach to healthcare provision, how the assumptions underpinning 'health' affect what is integral to a system and how this affects relationships between different stakeholders. Assuring both equity of access and safe, appropriate delivery of healthcare are viewed as essential goals.

DEFINING HEALTH

Our conceptual understanding of a health system is affected by which model of health is adopted. The biomedical model interprets health as the absence of disease or illness. The social model views health more broadly, adopting the World Health Organization's (WHO) Constitution of 1946, in which health is widely viewed as a state of complete physical, mental, and social well-being and not merely the absence of disease or infirmity.

While the biomedical definition interprets a health system as comprised of only the provision of healthcare services, a social definition includes social, economic, political and environmental factors that affect health and well-being. This chapter adopts the social definition of health.

WHAT IS A HEALTH SYSTEM?

Health systems can be defined as, 'organizations, institutions, and resources that deliver healthcare to individuals' (Mills and Ranson, 2012: 615). The most commonly used definition, however, is the WHO's (2000: xi), which defines a health system as, 'all the organizations, institutions and resources that are devoted to producing health actions [where a] health action is defined as any effort [...] whose primary purpose is to improve health'. These definitions distinguish between:

- health systems that have as their primary objective delivering quality, safe, accessible, affordable and equitable health services (such as antenatal visits for all pregnant mothers or treatment for tuberculosis)
- health systems that have as their primary objective improving health, which includes other health-related services (such as housing, education, clean water and sanitation).

These two definitions are related and a healthcare system can be seen as a part of the wider health system (Gerein et al., 2009).

The definitions of 'health' and 'health system' that one adopts ultimately affects the approaches and interventions used to strengthen the health system, but every health system has the following four objectives, with improving health being the main one (WHO, 2000, 2007):

1. improving the health of the population
2. being responsive to people's expectations
3. providing financial protection against the costs of ill health
4. improved efficiency.

These objectives are achieved through a combination of four interrelated functions:

1. providing health services (prevention, diagnosis, treatment and rehabilitation)
2. generating resources to spend on health (through taxation, for example)
3. financing health services to protect people against the costs of ill health and disability (through insurance, for example)
4. governing and regulating the health system, such as to ensure equal distribution of services (Skolnik, 2008).

Later in the chapter we discuss the question 'What is a health system?' in more detail.

HISTORY OF HEALTH SYSTEM DEVELOPMENT

This section introduces the history of national health systems' formation and development, key global health initiatives and the main international players.

HISTORY AND FORMATION OF NATIONAL HEALTH SYSTEMS

In low- and middle-income countries (LMICs), twentieth-century colonialism meant health services were concentrated in selected stations, available predominately to expatriates and the wealthy. Access to healthcare for the general public was often through missionary or religious organizations. The formation of national health systems effectively started following independence in African and Asian countries and, from the 1930s onwards, in Latin America. Postcolonial systems sought to overcome the inequitable and urban-concentrated services. Within many countries, due to a focus on curative services, this resulted in hospital-dominated health systems (Mills and Ranson, 2012).

PRIMARY HEALTHCARE MOVEMENT

The primary healthcare (PHC) movement attempted to reorientate the hospital-dominated focus of health systems. PHC was adopted at the 1978 joint WHO-UNICEF International Conference on Primary Healthcare, held at Alma-Ata, Soviet Union (the Alma-Ata Declaration). In this declaration, PHC is defined as, 'essential healthcare … made universally accessible to individuals and families' (WHO, 1978: 2). The declaration emphasized its five fundamental principles:

- equity
- health promotion and prevention
- community participation
- appropriate technology
- a multisectoral approach to health.

Robust PHC is a basis of any health system (see Chapter 8).

Implementation of PHC faced a number of challenges. The concept of a selective PHC was a response to rising costs and infrastructural constraints (Walsh and Warren, 1980). The idea behind selective PHC is that health systems can only afford to target specific areas of health – typically, those associated with high burdens of disease with effective low-cost interventions, such as GOBI FFF, which stands for growth monitoring, oral rehydration, breastfeeding, immunization, family spacing, food supplements and female education (WHO, 2005).

HEALTH REFORMS

The late 1980s and the early 1990s witnessed changes in the world's economy. Structural adjustment policies, promulgated by the International Monetary Fund and the World Bank, reflected a neo-liberal ideology and led to the decreasing role of governments in service provision. National health systems were criticized for failing to respond to health challenges, particularly the growing threat of HIV/AIDS. Poverty and inequality gaps widened, both within and between countries. Demographic transition and the rise in health costs resulted in acknowledging a close link between economics and health. Following the publication of the World Bank's World Development Report in 1993 calling for investment in health, economics was established as a dominant discipline within the health sector.

The 1980s and 1990s saw widespread health-sector reforms. The key components of the reforms were:

- involving the private sector and limiting the role of government to strategic direction through policymaking
- decentralization of authority over resource management from the centre to local levels
- regulation of public–private relationships to improve efficiency and equity
- improving health financing through introduction of user fees, community-based financing and different forms of health insurance (Mills and Ranson, 2012).

Health reforms highlighted the importance of a common platform for assessing and comparing countries' health systems. The publication of the World Health Report in 2000 by the WHO, although criticized for its methodology, marked the first attempt to assess and compare national health systems.

KEY GLOBAL HEALTH AGENDAS/INITIATIVES

After the Alma-Ata Declaration, in 1981 the WHO General Assembly unanimously adopted the 'Health for All' strategy to be achieved by the year 2000. This strategy emphasized two key aspects:

1. ensuring equity, that resources for health are evenly distributed and essential healthcare is accessible to everyone
2. prevention, that health is a responsibility of everyone and it is not just health staff who are to reduce the costs of curative care.

At the turn of the millennium, two international initiatives influenced health systems.

- The UN's Millennium Declaration, which defined the eight Millennium Development Goals (MDGs). They essentially represented commitments to reduce poverty and hunger and tackle ill health, gender disparity, lack of education, lack of access to clean water and environmental degradation.
- The Commission on Macroeconomics and Health – established by the WHO in January 2000 – submitted its report in December 2001. This was the first time since the World Development Report of 1993 that the relation between health and development was explicitly analyzed, informing a new strategy for investing in health for development.

Numerous programme-based international initiatives also emerged, such as:

- the WHO's 3 by 5 initiative, which, on World AIDS Day 2003, saw the WHO and UNAIDS set a target that three million people living with HIV/AIDS in developing countries would receive antiretroviral therapy by 2005
- the WHO's Global Malaria Programme, which provides advice and guidance to national malaria control programmes worldwide.

Within the last decade, a re-emergence of the PHC agenda has promoted universal health coverage (UHC), such as the WHO 2010 World Health Report. According to the WHO, the main goal of UHC is to ensure that all people can obtain health services without experiencing financial hardship. As with PHC, UHC is seen as a foundation of any health system.

MAIN INTERNATIONAL PLAYERS

Three groups of international players (or actors) influence national health systems:

- those with political influence
- those involved in funding health systems
- health service providers.

Activity 2.1

List the organizations you are aware of that influence national health systems. Start by considering your own country.

Comment

In terms of political influence, the global stage is dominated by two agencies: the WHO and the World Bank. The WHO was founded in 1948 as the UN's agency to lead and coordinate health activities globally, supported by its six regional and country offices (Walt et al., 2012). The political primacy of the WHO, associated with the PHC movement, diminished by the late 1980s and 1990s, when the World Bank became a major global health actor. By the late 1990s, however, the balance shifted again and the WHO regained its legitimacy, following the World Health Report 2000.

As for funding, international aid from industrialized countries is a major source of finance for LMICs' health systems. Donors can be bilateral (such as the USAID or the UK's DFID) or multilateral (the European Commission, for example). UN agencies also provide technical assistance for health systems or programmes, such as maternal and child health or HIV/AIDS control. Examples of these UN agencies include the WHO, United Nations Development Programme (UNDP), United Nations Population Fund (UNFPA) and United Nations Children's Fund (UNICEF) (Walt et al., 2012).

Private-sector finance is important for LMICs. Recent examples include major philanthropic institutions, such as the Bill & Melinda Gates Foundation, that funds HIV/AIDS treatment in African countries. Global public–private partnerships (for example, the global Vaccine Alliance – Gavi Alliance – and the Global Fund for AIDS, Malaria and TB) are also important. While these are set up as mechanisms for tapping funding for communicable disease control programmes, they can also divert resources away from neglected programmes (such as mental health).

As for service provision, health reforms stimulated international non-governmental organizations (INGOs), often referred to as civil society organisations (Walt et al., 2012). This led to the duplication and fragmentation of health services within many LMICs as donors sought to finance INGOs directly, bypassing the governments. While many INGOs were primarily established to deliver health services, nowadays they are increasingly involved in research, advocacy and even regulation.

UNDERSTANDING HEALTH SYSTEMS

In this section we examine how a 'health system' is defined and identify its key actors.

KEY APPROACHES TO UNDERSTANDING A HEALTH SYSTEM

Three perspectives on understanding health systems can be discerned.

1. The institutional or infrastructure model asks what structures work best to achieve health system objectives. For example, Kleczkowski et al. (1984) identified infrastructure (that is, health facilities and equipment) as central to ensuring healthcare delivery.
2. The economic model suggests that an adequate allocation and the best possible use of resources would achieve system goals (World Bank, 1993). It considers population needs, typically expressed in the form of consumer demands and health markets.
3. The function-based model emphasizes the relations between the four system functions and the four health system goals discussed earlier (WHO, 2007).

WHO BUILDING BLOCKS FRAMEWORK

In 2007, the WHO described six health systems building blocks that contribute to the achievement of its four goals of ensuring access, coverage, quality and safety of services (WHO, 2007):

1. the delivery of effective, safe, accessible, affordable, equitable health services of good quality that are responsive to the population's health needs
2. a well-functioning health workforce, comprised of doctors, nurses and other staff who are available, qualified and work responsively, fairly and efficiently
3. a robust health information system, ensuring reliable and timely information is produced, analyzed and disseminated for decisionmaking
4. appropriate and equitably distributed supply of medical products, vaccines and technologies to ensure quality healthcare
5. a good system for financing health that ensures people can afford the required services and are not impoverished by health costs
6. effective leadership and governance through an overseen regulated policy framework that addresses societal values such as equity.

Two points are worth emphasizing. First, each building block is complex. For example service delivery is comprised of different subsystems, such as quality assurance and patient referrals. Second, multiple relationships exist within and between the building blocks. For example, good governance requires leaders among the health workforce who have adequate information to inform their decisions.

More recently, the concepts of systems thinking and complex adaptive systems have been emphasized (de Savigny and Adam, 2009). This underlines two aspects of health systems:

- the systemic nature of health systems and the interdependency of the six building blocks, which revolve around people's needs
- the need for continuous adaptation and change of health systems to address a country's changing demographic and epidemiological profiles.

UNDERSTANDING DIFFERENCES BETWEEN HEALTH SYSTEMS

Different countries have different types of health systems. They can differ in the way that they are designed, how they are financed, the nature or degree of state intervention, the ownership and provision of services or how services are paid for (Mills and Ranson, 2012; Skolnik, 2008).

What is the evidence?

Key differences between health systems

Four types of health systems are described in the literature in relation to how health systems are financed and the role of the state (Table 2.1). In reality, however, health systems are complex and do not fall easily into one specific category.

Table 2.1   Key differences between health systems

Type/model	Public tax-based system	Public premium-financed system	Private insurance system	Mixed public and private systems
Example countries	United Kingdom Lesotho Swaziland	Germany Kenya	United States	India Hong Kong
Financed	Taxes.	Contributions from employers/ employees.	Privately financed.	Both public and private.
State intervention	Direct.	Mostly indirect.	Indirect.	Public, direct. Private, indirect.
Ownership of services	Public.	Public/private.	Mostly private.	Public/private.
Individual payment/ expenditure	Largely free at point of service, though out-of-pocket charges are common in LMICs.	Largely free at point of service.	Covered by insurance, but out-of-pocket charges for those without.	Public services mostly free at point of service, but private, largely out-of-pocket charges.
Overall quality	HIC – high to moderate. LMIC – mixed.	HIC – moderate to high. LMIC – mixed.	HIC – high.	HIC – high. LMIC – mixed (poor to high).
Regulation	HIC – high. LMIC – weak to moderate.	HIC – high.	HIC – moderate to high.	HIC – high. LIMIC – weak to moderate.

Source: Based on Skolnik (2008), Smith and Hanson (2012) and Stevens and Zee (2011)

Two caveats are appropriate in relation to health systems in LMICs: their resource-constrained nature and the related influence of international organizations. Within LMICs, external influences can have a particularly significant effect on how a health system is designed. Examples of these include the nature of postcolonial systems, available resources, past and current donor regulations and health reforms.

In addition, all health systems are affected by epidemiological and demographic trends. A country's burden of disease will also lead to different patterns of inequalities within a population, influencing which services are required and by whom.

KEY ACTORS WITHIN A NATIONAL HEALTH SYSTEM

Health systems are complex social institutions involving interactions between different actors, often with competing interests and agendas. There are four typical groups of actors within a country: the public sector, private sector, international agencies and its population.

─────────────────────── Activity 2.2 ───────────────────────

List the roles of the public sector at national, regional and local levels in your country. Afterwards compare your results with the information given in Table 2.2.

PUBLIC SECTOR

The public sector, including national and local governments, is a key player. Its role ranges from providing oversight and collaboration with other sectors through to healthcare delivery (Mills and Ranson, 2012). The public sector typically comprises three levels, carrying out different roles, as shown in Table 2.2.

Table 2.2 Typical roles of the public sector

Central/national	Region/province	District/local
Policymaking and planning.	Coordinating/bridging role between centre and district.	Assessing and prioritizing local issues.
Resource generation and allocation.	Strengthening of capacity of respective districts.	Promoting community participation and bottom-up planning processes.
Research and technology development.	Assisting districts in designing appropriate tools for supervision, monitoring and planning.	Implementing programmes and delivering services.
Operational responsibilities, such as the management of large hospitals.		

PRIVATE SECTOR

Earlier we referred to the private sector as being part of global public–private partnerships. Here we shall focus on the private sector at a country level.

Two types of private-sector actors exist: private for-profit and private not-for-profit (most commonly known as non-governmental organizations or NGOs). Private-sector tasks can include:

- policymaking and strategic planning
- research and advocacy
- financing healthcare
- provision of healthcare services.

Appropriate regulation of private-sector involvement is important, particularly where the private sector has the potential to grow and become an influential stakeholder.

INTERNATIONAL AGENCIES

Multilateral and bilateral aid agencies, and international and national NGOs, can play important roles in providing and channelling resources and placing health issues at the centre of international debates. International NGOs such as Oxfam or Save the Children can be synonymous with the private not-for-profit sector in relation to service delivery and advocacy for change. These are often in a better position to be autonomous partners as they are less influenced by a government's agenda than for-profit organizations. They can, however, also wish to safeguard their own autonomy and follow their own agendas, which can be detrimental to development. An NGO with a strong political or ethical agenda may push this agenda over the country's own priorities (such as an anti-abortion stance in relation to family planning).

THE POPULATION

Although a country's people are the main agents of their health, the role of the population is usually poorly recognized. The main role of the population is to help implement health programmes (through ensuring the attendance of children for immunization, for example). It is particularly important in relation to preventive services (such as ensuring healthy lifestyles) and in the uptake of primary care services (to reduce the risk of illness and thus reduce the costs of more expensive hospital care, for example). Better understanding of their role requires investigation on a range of questions, such as health-seeking behaviour, underlying reasons for practises, evaluation of needs and demands and underlying power structures within the society.

HEALTH SERVICE DELIVERY

Health service delivery is a central element of a health system, but it is only one of a number of interconnected systems components that have to work together. The degree to which health services are effective, safe and of good quality depends on the other system components.

----------------------------------- Activity 2.3 -----------------------------------

List some factors that you consider important in ensuring that health services are effective.

Comment

Effective health services require available and trained staff, adequate infrastructure, appropriate medicine and working equipment. Furthermore, appropriate regulatory mechanisms are needed to ensure that incentives are offered for both service providers and users (WHO, 2007).

Six questions are important with regard to healthcare delivery within LMICs (Gerein et al., 2009).

1. What types of services are needed and at what level?
2. Where should services be provided?
3. What relationships should exist between these services?
4. Who owns/provides these services?
5. How should quality be maintained?
6. How do we ensure an appropriate level of access and equity?

Each of these is explored below.

WHAT TYPES OF SERVICES ARE NEEDED AND AT WHAT LEVEL?

The levels of healthcare are as follows (Gerein et al., 2009; Skolnik, 2008).

1. **Primary healthcare (PHC)** The first point of contact, offering generalized as opposed to specialized care. It is provided at the grass roots or community level and consists of a basic or essential package of health services, including facility-based outpatient and outreach services within the community. PHC centres often act as gatekeepers to secondary facilities, referring patients based on need.
2. **Secondary healthcare** Specialized care provided within local or district hospitals. It often consists of specialist diagnostic facilities and expertise and includes outpatient and inpatient services.
3. **Tertiary healthcare** Highly specialized care provided in regional or national hospitals after referral from secondary healthcare facilities. This is the most sophisticated and resource-intensive level of services.

Services provided at each level are not always exclusive to that level. For example, some primary healthcare services can also be provided through the outpatient clinics at hospitals. In addition, while primary healthcare often acts as a gateway to secondary healthcare, and secondary care a gateway to tertiary healthcare, this is not always the case. In China, for example, primary healthcare practitioners do not act as gatekeepers to district hospitals and individuals are able to choose which level is their first port of call. This can also be the case in countries that have a large private sector, such as India.

Activity 2.4

What types of health services exist within a health system? List services that could be offered for a national tuberculosis (TB) control programme. Afterwards, review Table 2.3 for examples of TB control services.

Three types of health services exist: promotive, preventive and curative services (see Table 2.3).

Table 2.3   Examples of services for a TB control programme

Types of services	Examples of services
Promotive aimed at promoting an appropriate lifestyle to avoid exposure to harmful factors leading to a disease.	Campaign against smoking.
Preventive aimed at preventing the development of a disease.	Vaccination against TB.
Curative aimed at treating the disease, such as prescribing medicines or carrying out surgical operations.	Prescription of antibiotics and observing daily intake by staff.

The types of services provided and at which level depends on a country's disease burden, priorities and availability of resources.

WHERE SHOULD SERVICES BE PROVIDED?

The location of health services affects access to health facilities, influencing health equity within a country. According to Gerein et al. (2009: 87), decisions regarding health service location should be based on factors including, 'health needs, population densities, the transportation infrastructure, and the relative costs of the service'.

Within LMICs most health facilities are found within urban areas, leaving rural areas underserved. This is often due to a difference in rural–urban distribution of qualified health workers, leaving rural areas significantly disadvantaged. Outreach services support clinics to reach underserved areas, with health workers travelling to provide essential services such as health education and immunization (Gerein et al., 2009).

WHAT RELATIONSHIPS SHOULD EXIST BETWEEN THESE SERVICES?

Important relationships exist between services. For example, patients should be able to move between primary, secondary, and tertiary levels as needed and with ease, or receive a combination of services at the same level. Patients' movement across the levels relates to processes of referral between the different levels, known as vertical integration, whereas the latter relates to referral between different services or programmes at the same level (or the receipt of different services at the same level), known as horizontal integration (Gerein et al., 2009). With horizontal integration, an HIV positive patient might receive antiretroviral therapy

(ART), tuberculosis medication and advice on malaria prevention within one visit to a healthcare centre. Vertical integration is important to ensure a well-functioning healthcare system where services are provided at multiple levels. It requires a clear understanding of roles and responsibilities at each level, lines of communication, adequate transportation, especially for emergency situations, and feedback systems between the different levels.

Non-integrated services (or programmes) are those that only offer one type of service, such as ART for HIV positive patients or TB treatment. Non-integrated services can allow for a clear technical focus, specialization and prioritization of a particular health problem through earmarked funding. Integrated services, however, allow for better management of health services and greater opportunities for maintaining and improving health more generally.

WHO OWNS/PROVIDES THESE SERVICES?

Mills and Ranson (2012: 638) identify seven categories of healthcare providers in LMICs:

1. state-run health providers
2. social insurance agencies running services for the insured and their dependants
3. civil society organizations (CSOs), including faith-based organizations (FBOs) and NGOs
4. occupational healthcare providers
5. private for-profit providers
6. traditional providers
7. informal sector providers, including drug pedlars.

Although the public sector may predominate in many high-income societies, within LMICs, the private, civil society and informal or traditional sectors play a significant role in healthcare provision (Mills and Ranson, 2012). Where public services are insufficient or do not exist, the state can also contract in services from private and CSO providers. Secondary or tertiary hospitals will often be run by private or CSO providers, but will be contracted by the public sector.

HOW SHOULD QUALITY BE MAINTAINED?

Maintaining the quality of health services is an important consideration, and challenge, in many countries. Common quality problems include: poorly trained or unmotivated staff, poor management, inadequate infrastructure and lack of medical equipment or supplies. How patients perceive quality is an important determinant in their selection of healthcare providers. In many LMICs, the public sector is often – and sometimes wrongly – perceived as low quality when it comes to the issues of responsiveness of staff, consultation time, privacy, likelihood of receiving information about diagnosis and prognosis and overall patient diagnosis. This perception often pushes many patients to the private sector, which has higher out-of-pocket expenditures.

In reality, however, the actual quality of public providers can be higher than that of private providers when it comes to issues such as adherence to medical management standards or prescription guidelines, knowledge and understanding of correct diagnosis and treatment, diagnostic accuracy, incidence of unnecessary and expensive procedures and emphasis on preventive care. Quality assurance is therefore important, requiring effective governance and regulation of health systems.

Activity 2.5

List factors improving the quality of health services.

Comment

Quality assurance mechanisms include developing quality objectives, communicating set standards to health facilities and health professionals, developing indicators and monitoring facilities. They therefore require the development and enforcement of incentives for compliance and sanctions for non-compliance – something that many LMICs do not have the capacity to do.

HOW DO WE ENSURE AN APPROPRIATE LEVEL OF ACCESS AND EQUITY?

Health disparities are a common feature of many health systems within LMICs. Lower socio-economic groups, those living in rural areas and specific cultural or disadvantaged groups can lack access to even basic health services. It is important to ensure that all population groups have equitable access to at least essential health services. In particular, the cost of healthcare can be inaccessible to many groups and poorer families can find themselves faced with catastrophic health expenditures when a family member falls ill. The push towards universal health coverage, discussed above, is one way to address this. Other strategies include community health insurance schemes and subsidized services for disadvantaged groups (Skolnik, 2008).

What is the evidence?

Examples of healthcare systems

The healthcare system in Tanzania

Tanzania's healthcare system is largely publicly provided and, for many years, only a limited number of private for-profit facilities existed. This is partly due to private health services being banned after independence. In 1991, however, the development of private health facilities was permitted with approval from the Ministry of Health and Social Welfare (MOHSW). The current healthcare system is predominately financed by general tax revenue and donor

(Continued)

(Continued)

funding. Out-of-pocket payments contribute a significant proportion of total healthcare costs, constituting over half of household contributions to healthcare. Health insurance covers less than 10 per cent of the population.

The use of traditional health services is high and the MOHSW estimated in 2007 that 60 per cent of all those seeking healthcare depend on some form of these services (Kwesigaboa et al., 2012). Like many LMICs, the public healthcare system has several levels. The levels include village health services, dispensary services (serving 6000 to 10,000 people), health centre services (serving 50,000 people), district hospitals, regional hospitals and four tertiary hospitals. Where possible, hospitals are publically provided, but the government also contracts NGO-run hospitals (Government of Tanzania, 2013; Skolnik, 2008).

The healthcare system in India

India has a mixed healthcare system. Despite a large public healthcare network, public spending on health remains very low, at about 1 per cent of gross domestic product (GDP) (Peters et al., 2002). This has led to large private out-of-pocket health expenditures – approximately 80 per cent of all healthcare expenditures (Kumar et al., 2011). Health insurance coverage is limited, with approximately 10 per cent of the population covered (Kumar et al., 2011).

India has a tiered network of public health services. This includes health subcentres (serving 3000 to 5000 people), primary health centres (serving 20,000 to 30,000 people), community health centres (serving 80,000 to 120,000 people) and hospitals (Skolnik, 2008). Traditional practitioners are an important group of providers, too, with many people seeking care from traditional health services.

While health is a shared responsibility of central government and the states, many policy choices are devolved to the states, leading to large variations in healthcare provision and quality (Peters et al., 2002).

APPROACHES TO STRENGTHENING HEALTH SYSTEMS AND FUTURE DEVELOPMENT

In this final section, we summarize the key approaches to strengthening health systems and ask if we are now entering a new phase in their development.

APPROACHES TO STRENGTHENING HEALTH SYSTEMS

A major issue during the last 20 years has been finding an adequate balance between the so-called 'horizontal' and 'vertical' approaches. The debate continues. Vertical approaches include national programmes targeted at particular diseases, whereas horizontal approaches involve a PHC-orientated integrated approach. Policy decisions should be informed by evidence on which approaches are most effective within a particular context. This debate represents an opportunity to generate such evidence and inform policy choices.

The approaches to strengthening health systems include the following.

- PHC-based approaches emphasizing preventive and grass roots services as opposed to more curative and hospital-based care. They promote equity and universal access to health services.
- Neo-liberal approaches emphasizing use of markets within health systems, opposing centrally planned, more controlled health systems. They promote competition and individual choice regarding service providers.
- Focusing on selected attributes, whether a building block (such as human resource management) or a specific programme (such as maternal and child health or TB control) as opposed to more holistic, horizontal approaches. It assumes that changes such as improvements in service outcomes are more realistic within a single programme and on a small scale.

THE FUTURE OF HEALTH SYSTEMS DEVELOPMENT

Approaches to health reforms, initiated in the 1990s, have seen many changes:

- A softening of a strict market or neo-liberal approach in some international agencies. There is a renewed interest in overcoming poverty.
- Reduction in financing and conducting separate projects in developing countries, with a move towards operating through more established NGO and government structures. In some respects, this is expressed through budget support and Sector Wide Approaches (SWAps).
- Recognition that contemporary health-sector reform has focused on finance and organization of the health sector, but underemphasized the important issues of equity and human resources for health.
- Critical questions about the appropriateness of health-sector reforms, such as user fees, private contracting and decentralization, supported by research, prompt a more cautious approach.

Thus, increasing attention is being paid to the following five aspects of strengthening health systems, which provides an agenda for the next decade.

First, develop capacity within the whole health sector at three levels:

- individual skills and competencies
- organizational arrangements, such as adequate distribution of tasks and clear job descriptions
- system-wide attributes, such as appropriate resource environment and political commitment.

Second, focus on more 'holistic' development of health systems, to ensure sustainability. Given that there is no one single determinant of a well-functioning health system, there is a need to recognize the complex relations between the different health system components (de Savigny and Adam, 2009). Promoting effective bureaucracies and institutions, innovation and resilience are emphasized, in addition to more 'conventional' elements, such as effective leadership and governance, effective resource management and robust information systems (Balabanova et al., 2013).

Third, link disease control to changes in health systems. The conventional project-based approach is likely to continue, at least for globally prevalent diseases such as TB, HIV/AIDS and malaria. There is an increasing recognition, however, that health programmes do not work in isolation – they influence, or are influenced by, other health programmes. For example, strengthening individual skills of PHC staff in TB control, while it will improve the identification of TB cases, will leave less time for them to devote to antenatal care and other duties.

Fourth, develop more evidence-informed decisionmaking. Rational health policy, planning and management decisions informed by timely and reliable evidence are increasingly promoted nationally and internationally. Establishing research policy partnerships and strengthening the role of health systems and policy research generates such evidence.

Finally, renew interest in equity, as part of the agenda for UHC. The calls for UHC were part of the Alma-Ata Declaration. Many countries, following numerous health reforms, recognized the importance of PHC services and ensuring health equity. Knowledge about effective strategies to achieve UHC within different contexts is growing.

CONCLUSION

This chapter introduced the health system, its historical development, its organization, its composition, the key actors involved and the main approaches to strengthening health systems. Five aspects of strengthening health systems provide an agenda for the future.

REFERENCES

Balabanova, D., Mills, A., Conteh, L., Akkazieva, B., Banteyerga, H., Dash, U. et al. (2013) 'Good health at low cost 25 years on: lessons for the future of health systems strengthening', *The Lancet*, 381: 2118–2133.

de Savigny, D. and Adam, T. (eds) (2009) *Systems Thinking for Health Systems Strengthening*. Geneva: Alliance for Health Policy and Systems Research, World Health Organization.

Gerein, N., Green, A., Mirzoev, T. and Pearson, S. (2009) 'Health system impacts on maternal and child health'. In J. Ehiri and M. Meremikwu (eds), *International Maternal and Child Health*. Washington, DC: Springer Publishers.

Government of Tanzania (2013) *Health* [Online]. Available at: www.tanzania.go.tz/home/pages/16 (accessed 21 October 2013).

Kleczkowski, B.M., Roemer, M.I. and Werff, A.v.d. (1984) *National Health Systems and their Reorientation Towards Health For All: Guidelines For Policy-making*. Geneva: World Health Organization.

Kumar, A., Chen, L., Choudhury, M., Ganju, S., Mahajan, V., Sinha, A. et al. (2011) 'Financing healthcare for all: challenges and opportunities', *The Lancet*, 377: 668–679.

Kwesigaboa, G., Mwangua, M., Kakokoa, D., Warrinerb, I., Mkonyc, C., Killewoa, J. et al. (2012) 'Tanzania's health system and workforce crisis', *Journal of Public Health Policy*, 33: S35–S44.

Mills, A. and Ranson, K. (2012) 'The design of health systems'. In M.H. Merson, R.E. Black and A.J. Mills (eds), *Global Health. Diseases, Programs, Systems, and Policies*, 3rd edition. Burlington, USA: Jones and Bartlett Publishers, Inc.

Peters, D., Yazbeck, A., Sharma, R., Ramana, G., Pritchett, L. and Wagstaff, A. (2002) *Better Health Systems for India's Poor: Findings, Analysis, and Options*. Washington, DC: The World Bank.

Skolnik, R. (2008) An *Introduction to Health Systems. Essentials of Global Health*. Sudbury: Jones & Bartlett Learning.

Smith, R. and Hanson, K. (eds) (2012) *Health Systems in Low- and Middle-Income Countries*. Oxford: Oxford University Press.

Stevens, F. and Zee, J. (2011) 'Health system organization models (including targets and goals for health systems)'. In G. Carrin, K. Buse, H. Heggenhougen and S. Quah (eds), *Health Systems Policy, Finance and Organization*. Oxford: Elsevier.

Walsh, J. and Warren, K. (1980) 'Selective primary healthcare: an interim strategy for disease control in developing countries', *Social Science & Medicine*, 14: 145–163.

Walt, G., Buse, K. and Harmer, A. (2012) 'Cooperation in global health'. In M.H. Merson, R.E. Black and A.J. Mills (eds), *Global Health. Diseases, Programs, Systems, and Policies*, 3rd edition. Burlington, USA: Jones and Bartlett Publishers, Inc.

WHO (1978) *Declaration of Alma-Ata, Alma Ata*. USSR: World Health Organization, UNICEF, World Bank.

WHO (2000) *The World Health Report 2000. Health Systems: Improving Performance*. Geneva: World Health Organization.

WHO (2005) *World Health Report. Chapter 5: Choosing Interventions to Reduce Specific Risks*. Geneva: World Health Organization.

WHO (2007) *Everybody's Business: Strengthening Health Systems to Improve Health Outcomes: WHO's Framework For Action*. Geneva: World Health Organization.

World Bank (1993) *World Development Report: Investing in Health*. Washington, DC: World Bank.

HUMAN RESOURCES FOR HEALTH

ANN K. ALLEN AND JUDY MCKIMM

Chapter overview

After reading this chapter you will be able to:

- explain what human resources are needed to improve global health
- identify socio-economic and other factors affecting access to trained healthcare workers
- explain how to match workforce production to population needs and expectations
- assess factors involved in deploying, retaining and managing a health workforce
- evaluate policies to improve access to and the performance of healthcare
- explain what is involved in building capacity in human resources for health.

INTRODUCTION

Although matters have improved since the 2006 WHO report alerted us to the importance of building workforce capacity in order to achieve the Millennium Development Goals (MDGs), it is estimated that by 2035, there will be a global deficit of 12.9 million skilled health workers – that is, professionally trained nurses, doctors and midwives (WHO/WWA, 2014). Providing universal health coverage (UHC), 'based on an adequate, skilled, well-trained and motivated workforce', equitably, is now a political imperative in a global and urbanized economy (Campbell et al., 2013; UN, 2012; WHO, n.d.). A contributory factor to the short-fall of skilled personnel in low-income countries has been the exodus of trained health workers to meet the needs of wealthier economies, drawn by better pay and working conditions. This has encouraged innovative approaches to extend health practitioner roles (McKimm et al., 2013).

Expanding and ageing populations create new challenges that the health systems of LMICs are ill equipped to meet and some high-income countries are also struggling to sustain universal health coverage. The fiscal constraints imposed by austerity measures to address economic recession leave no country untouched and the growing burden of long-term conditions exacerbates existing demands generated by infectious diseases and the need for obstetric care.

Following the WHO report (2006), a Global Health Workforce Alliance (GHWA) was launched and, in 2010, the World Health Assembly agreed a code of practice on health workers' recruitment internationally (WHO, 2010). In 2012, a UN resolution, 'urged member states to develop health systems that avoid substantial direct payments at the point of delivery and to implement mechanisms for pooling risks to avoid catastrophic healthcare spending and impoverishment. This resolution sets the stage for UHC to become a unifying central health goal in the post-2015 Millennium Development Goal framework' (Vega, 2013: 179). Global consultation regarding the sustainable goals for health post 2015 conducted from September 2012 stated that, 'the health community needs to articulate, confidently but clearly, the contribution of health to sustainable development (Berkley et al., 2013), and acknowledge the crucial importance of the determinants of health by adopting a health-in-all-policies approach, recognizing the contributions of other sectors and setting health-related targets under other goals' (Task Team, 2013: 1443).

This chapter explains how managing to do more with the limited resources available globally will require a paradigm shift in how healthcare provision is made. Well-resourced countries can learn from the use of skills mix innovations generated by the needs of LMICs, such as task shifting, that, in turn, can benefit from the lessons of health promotion and the advances made in the use of mobile technology in industrialized societies. Today, it is not enough to consider only the numbers of health workers available in a health system; considerations such as accessibility, their acceptability to service users, the quality of the service provided and standards of performance are also important. Health workers should not be seen merely as health system inputs.

As individuals respond to both positive and negative motivating factors, ensuring best performance requires supportive management and safe, conducive practice environments. Training of clinicians should enhance their ability to act as change agents because they are well positioned to know what is needed at the front line. Health professionals decide point-of-service treatment, so their actions determine how efficiently other resources are used. Dynamic forecasting models, informed by labour market analyses as well as being responsive to the demands created by the specific epidemiological needs of different locations and populations, are needed. It is important to respond to the complex and adaptive entities that healthcare systems and the health workforce are. Thus, trained and adequately supported human resource managers must be part of the labour force of health systems at all levels.

THE LABOUR FORCE OF A HEALTHCARE SYSTEM

This section discusses which occupations contribute to improving the health of populations and the qualities needed at both system and individual levels. Factors that constrain the efficient delivery of safe, appropriate, high-quality care are discussed. In Chapter 2 we discussed the distinction between biomedical and social models of health. Adopting one of these models in preference to the other has implications for how the boundaries of health systems are defined. This chapter assumes a social definition of health.

---------------------------------- Activity 3.1 ----------------------------------

List the occupations important for an effective health system.

Comment

You will probably have included doctors, nurses, midwives and managers on your list. Did you also think of groups such as community health workers (CHWs), pharmacists, laboratory technicians, logistics managers, drivers, porters, security guards, environmental health workers, nutritionists, veterinary surgeons …? 'The health workforce consists of all people engaged in actions whose primary intent is to improve health. This includes health service providers, such as doctors, nurses, midwives, pharmacists and community health workers. It also includes health management and support workers, such as hospital administrators, district health managers and social workers, who dedicate all or part of their time to improving health' (WHO/GWA, 2014 www.who.int/hrh/workforce_mdgs/en/)

The delivery of safe healthcare requires inputs from a variety of staff with different skills and levels of education, but their ability to perform is also affected by factors in other sectors, such as:

- legislation that prevents some staff from being trained to do tasks associated with other professional groups or the use of drugs that have not been certified
- privileging some communities with respect to roadbuilding or infrastructure, thereby restricting access and leading to deprivation
- decisions being made in one sector without regard for the impact on others (as when commercial production for foreign exchange ousts subsistence farming in marginal lands).

Adopting a 'health-in-all-policies' approach by a government means that the potential adverse consequences on health of decisions made in sectors outside its ministry of health can be mitigated.

INADEQUATE STAFFING PROVISION

LMICs fall far short of the WHO recommended ratios for trained clinical staff: 'Only 5 of the 49 countries categorized as low-income economies by the World Bank meet the minimum threshold of 23 doctors, nurses and midwives per 10,000 population that was established by WHO as necessary to deliver essential maternal and child health services' (WHO/GWA, 2014). Further, 'Sub-Saharan Africa has only 2 doctors and 11 nurses or midwives per 10,000 people, compared with approximately 30 physicians and 84 nurses or midwives per 10,000 people in high-income countries' (Silvestri et al., 2014: 750). These critical shortages, alongside unequal geographical distribution and frequently an inadequate mix of skills, mean that the poor – particularly in rural areas remote from cities – have little access to allopathic medicine. Consequently, they are very vulnerable to infectious disease outbreaks, such as cholera, typhoid and Ebola.

Case study   Ebola and the need for skilled and properly resourced staff

In 2014, a number of West African countries experienced outbreaks of Ebola haemorrhagic fever. This highly infectious disease (first identified in 1976 in Zaire – now the Democratic Republic of Congo – and Southern Sudan) has an extremely high fatality rate and patients need to be treated in isolation by staff wearing protective clothing and practising impeccable hygiene. It is transmitted through close contact with blood, secretions or other bodily fluids.

Terrified communities resisted going to clinics for treatment in the early stages when it might have been possible to treat them successfully because they believed health workers were causing the disease. In countries such as Guinea, Liberia and Sierra Leone, people were highly exposed to the risk of transmission because of inadequate water and sanitation and most people having little education. Customs such as bush meat consumption and mourning deceased relatives by having direct contact with their cadavers increased the risk of infection.

24.03.2014

An outbreak of Ebola haemorrhagic fever in southern Guinea has prompted the international medical organisation Médecins Sans Frontières/Doctors Without Borders (MSF) to launch an emergency response.

Twenty-four MSF doctors, nurses, logisticians and hygiene and sanitation experts are already in the country, while additional staff will strengthen the team in the coming days.

www.msf.org.uk/article/guinea-ebola-epidemic-declared

By August 2014, the WHO, recognizing the outbreak as an international health emergency, issued recommendations, including the adoption of exceptional regulatory procedures. At the request of the governments of affected countries, the United States and UK sent military personnel to help contain the disease, engineers to build clinics and install utilities, equipment and trained staff, plus protective clothing. Alongside this aid, scientists collaborated internationally to produce drugs and a vaccine for a disease that for 40 years had not been prioritized.

Workers acting in a health system are very diverse, not limited to professionals providing frontline care. Although national governments are responsible for setting the parameters of routine health services (whether delivered publicly, privately or in a mixed economy of care), health issues that cross country/regional boundaries often require a global, international response.

Note that adopting exceptional regulatory procedures enabled untested drugs to be used for a few infected people flown to America or Europe for treatment. More significantly, acting in this way spurred international collaboration to develop a vaccine by reducing the time required for it to be field-tested.

———————————————— Activity 3.2 ————————————————

Identify reasons for external support being needed to address the Ebola epidemic.

Comment

We expect you thought about poverty, as well as lack of staff and equipment to protect health workers because of weak and under-resourced health systems. Dr Bintu Mansaray, posted to help the Ministry of Health and Sanitation, Sierra Leone, describes the reality of working conditions for local workers (HIFA2015, 2014):

> As a medical doctor currently working in Sierra Leone I just shake my head at the outrageous comments people make. We're fighting a disease we new [knew] nothing about. I had a one page note on Ebola whilst in medical school in Sierra Leone bcos (sic) it wasn't endemic to my region instead we extensively studied Lassa Fever, Yellow Fever, Rabies etc. under haemorrhagic fevers. Nurses never even heard the word Ebola so for some people to be blaming health personnel who are dying that we're being careless is heartrending. Av (sic) lost colleagues and friends to this fight that has no end in sight. We work in hospitals with no running water. We tell people about handwashing when they get their water from streams. We have patients coming into the hospitals lying about their symptoms. Everyone now knows the symptoms of Ebola and they carefully deny each one. But in Sierra Leone we're still working. The things we've seen and are still seeing just breaks my heart. You wear a PPE and in an hour ure (sic) sweating like ure in hell. Uve (sic) got 50–80 patients to check on and by the time ure on patient 20 you can no longer breath in that PPE. Ebola is a scourge that should soon be eradicated. My prayer is on the vaccine. In Sierra Leone we have 136 doctors for about 6 million people. 5 are dead. All we depend on now is on international help. We need health personnel. The more health workers in treatment centers the less often health workers enter into the treatment tents, thus lowering the risk of infection. Organizations like Doctors Without Borders and Emergency Surgical Centre has been such tremendous help there's no way the people of our countries can say thank you. I am pleading for more health personnel. My people are suffering and dying and such helplessness we feel is psychologically daunting.

Migration of health professionals from LMICs to better-resourced countries and the preference of people to move to urban areas where living conditions better suit their needs than do rural areas, make for inequitable distributions of health workers globally, regionally and nationally. Frontline workers providing clinical care need to be responsive to the needs of the population they serve, which means they need to be properly trained, supervised and supported by the health system. 'Health services should be organized and delivered to be comprehensive, integrated and people-centred to increase access to healthcare in rural and remote areas. A greater focus is required on putting incentives in place and ensuring good working conditions that can enhance health workforce productivity, quality and responsiveness. Bringing about lasting change in human resources for health requires the collaboration of sectors and constituencies' (WHO/GWA, 2014: vii).

CONSTRAINTS ON PROVISION OF THE WORKFORCE REQUIRED

Clinically trained professionals are vital for any healthcare system. The WHO standard for developing countries in respect of physicians is 1:10,000 people. Producing the number of health workers needed to provide access to care for the whole population is a major challenge.

For instance, in Ethiopia, where there was one physician for every 100,000 people (and a considerably worse ratio in some remote parts of the country), the need to train more doctors led to the establishment of 13 new medical schools in 2012. A high annual attrition rate, fast population growth, the expansion of both governmental and non-governmental health institutions and the limited number of medical school places explained the extremely low physician-to-population ratio in Ethiopia (Berhan, 2008).

Medical school expansion more than doubled the number of student places. Yet, equipping these medical schools with clinical teachers is constrained by clinicians' availability, salary costs and the opportunity costs of service provision as their time is taken up with teaching, examining and the administrative tasks associated with university education. Few incentives exist for senior doctors to teach in medical schools, which means newly graduated doctors with limited experience are recruited to teach and administer the new schools.

Benchmarking higher education performance so as to protect standards is costly and also can be perceived as challenging the tradition of academic autonomy. Many doctors leave Ethiopia for higher-paying jobs overseas and those who stay tend to work in the cities and in the private sector. Unless salaries and employment conditions are improved, medically qualified academic staff may not be recruited or retained. Benefitting one group of academics without improving the employment conditions of other academics involved in medical education, such as scientists and social scientists, may be difficult and, thus, add to the costs of educational provision. Scaling up enrolment can also affect the students' learning experience.

Dame Endalew, a medical student at St Paul's, says the sharp increase in enrolment has made it difficult to learn.

'There's a scarcity of resources,' Endalew said. 'We don't have books, computer labs, lecturers. Every time the number of students increases, these things become worsened.'

He says he often can't complete assignments because all of the books and computers are in use. He had to share a cadaver with 30 peers. And he often interviews patients who have already seen 10 or 15 other medical students.

'When you try to work with them, they are really fed up with the students asking the same question again and again,' he said.

www.pri.org/stories/2012-12-20/ethiopias-crowded-medical-schools

---

Training sufficient numbers of health workers involves making changes in higher education institutions that may be resisted. The assumptions and values of academics and health professionals frequently differ. Ideas of 'academic freedom' do not sit comfortably with being told what to teach, although this may be mitigated by financial inducements. Knowledge production is rated by academics more highly than knowledge transmission for use. Traditionally, many higher education institutions have valued 'education' over 'training'. Education is perceived as transformative, with the aim of creating independent and creative individuals willing to challenge existing mores. Training, however, is viewed as an instrumental activity, aimed at creating a competent workforce to serve the economic goals of effectiveness and efficiency. Over time the distinctions may blur as universities add 'service to the wider community' as an approved goal in their mission statements.

Even when large numbers of students are trained, however, they may not remain in their health workforce. Data from a multicountry cross-sectional survey of 3199 first- and final-year medical and nursing students at 16 premier government institutions in Bangladesh, Ethiopia, India, Kenya, Malawi, Nepal, the United Republic of Tanzania and Zambia, 'suggest that in nations with critical shortages of health professionals, nearly a quarter of medical students and over a third of nursing students surveyed felt very likely to leave their country within five years post-training. Meanwhile, less than one fifth of students anticipated a rural career. Much of this intent appears suggested by characteristics evident even before enrolment' (Silvestri et al., 2014: 753).

Migration is complex – it involves more than a simple loss or gain of individual workers. While health workforce migration may be problematic for a country or region, the communities or families left behind often benefit from (even survive as a result of) income sent back 'home' by the health worker who has moved to a higher-income country. Such 'remission' helps families remain in their local communities (which benefits such communities) even though, from a national workforce perspective, there has been a net loss of those workers. In many regions of the world (the Pacific, north-western Europe, Africa, Indian subcontinent, the Caribbean), such labour migration is part of a 'diaspora' – a scattering or dispersion of peoples to other parts of the region or world, who retain a practical, financial and psychological attachment to their ancestral home.

MEETING HEALTH NEEDS IN RURAL AND REMOTE POPULATIONS

While we are rapidly moving towards a world where mega-cities grow upwards and outwards, many areas of the world are remote and rural. Mountainous terrain, as in the Andes and the Himalayas, tracts of desert or dispersed island communities may be sparsely inhabited and land that is agriculturally productive, forested or pastured may also have low population densities. Provision of healthcare in such rural or remote areas, whatever the income of the country, requires the adoption of different models:

> The Regional strategy on human resources for health 2006–2015, developed by the WHO Regional Office for the Western Pacific (WHO, 2007) identifies the need to 'enable the delivery of effective health services by addressing workforce size, distribution and skill mix' as one of five key strategic objectives. More specifically, it seeks a key outcome where 'effective strategies are in place to minimize distribution imbalances', with a focus on 'workforce requirements and incentives to work in underserved and rural/remote areas', including use of incentives, supportive supervision and multipurpose workers.' (Buchan et al., 2011: 2)

Activity 3.3

Read Buchan et al. (2011) (available online at: http://whqlibdoc.who.int/publications/2011/9789241501255_eng.pdf?ua=1).
   What helps to retain staff in remote and rural areas?

Comment

Appointment of health workers who come originally from the area to which they are deployed means they retain extended family connections and are familiar with local customs and language. For this reason, in Ethiopia, where 80 per cent of the population are unlikely to see a doctor because of the remote and mountainous areas in which they live, the policy is to appoint local women to be village health workers. They are chosen by their communities and trained and supported to provide basic care and health education by healthcare workers based in clinics but doing outreach work.

   Providing incentives (such as financial, housing, healthcare benefits) may be sufficient inducement for nurse practitioners to remain in post. Extending nurses' scope of practice is a tried and tested way throughout the world of providing healthcare where there is a shortage of doctors who may be reluctant to work outside urban areas. For higher-level skills and clinical procedures, mobile teams and the use of mobile technologies are valuable.

WORKFORCE PLANNING

Workforce planning estimates health workforce requirements based on a country's epidemiological and demographic profile, then scaling up education and training capacities to narrow the gap between the required number of health workers and the existing number (McPake et al., 2013).

   In many countries, once students have become accredited professionals, it is usually a matter of individual choice where they will seek work. In some countries, however, health professionals are indentured or bonded to work for a certain length of time in their own country, sometimes in rural areas, as part of national service.

   You have already seen that opportunities for skilled professionals are global. A health system needs continuously to recruit, deploy and retain staff by attending to factors such as salary, working conditions and opportunities for development. It also needs to replace those lost to retirement, resignations and migration. Workers need to routinely update their skills and knowledge and so supervision and performance monitoring are also needed to ensure the quality of care provided. All these factors affecting motivation and performance need to be planned for and supported. Planning for the future requires forecasting population needs in relation to the predicted health and disease burden and identifying workforce training and retention targets.

   At the organizational level, matching human resources with current and future activities can be problematic. Management must forecast the demand and supply of human resources as part of the organization's functional planning processes. Forecasting estimates future labour availability and needs.

———————————————————— **Activity 3.4** ————————————————————

Do you think forecasts are the same as plans or targets? If not, explain your reasoning.

Comment

If you said, 'Yes', it's perhaps because the words are often used interchangeably. In fact they do refer to different things.

Plans are tools used to achieve a desired result. Targets, goals or objectives are the specific results you want to achieve. Planning is a process of establishing objectives and courses of action prior to taking action. It is a comprehensive framework for making decisions in advance. Planning includes forecasting, along with establishing the timeframe and activities needed to build workforce capacity.

Planning workforce numbers and the mix of professions and specialties needed may be based on norms set by governments (often based on historical practice) or, where administrative records are reliably kept and analyses of the data conducted, it is possible to take a more predictive approach.

Workload indicators of staffing need (WISN), a forecasting model favoured by the WHO, acknowledges that staffing requirements vary among health facilities based on the consideration of workloads. Other methods of forecasting use fixed ratios (population or bed ratio) or standardized service levels by facility type. Traditionally, setting staff levels in health facilities by using population ratios (such as doctors, nurses, health officers) per 1000 patients has been used. This helps in estimating overall staff requirements, setting standard staffing schedules (staff allocated to each health post, health centre and district hospital, for example) and the training loads for health services in the facilities concerned.

While staff norms may help managers with planning services, because of their general nature, they may not actually reflect the complexity of a specific context.

Most norms make explicit or implicit assumptions about the numbers of hours people will work, the amount of leave they will take (sickness, holidays or special leave for training) and the patterns of care that will be delivered. Particular groups of workers will be deemed to have a particular role to play in the delivery of healthcare.

There are different types of norms.

- **The 'ideal service' norm** The staffing patterns envisaged in this type of indicator may not be achieved for many years and no realistic target date can be set. When norms fall into this category, planners have to consider what intermediate targets should be aimed for by a known date. This allows the human resources structure to evolve smoothly and types of staff appropriate to the eventual pattern are not recruited in advance of the pace of development of the service.
- **The 'policy' norms** Staffing levels are set at a particular level – or X per cent above the present level – because agreed policy is to develop services within the area. These norms will usually have a target date and progress towards them should be monitored. For example, a policy norm may be to say that, because primary care services in primary hospitals are being expanded, in five years' time an additional 30 per cent of primary hospitals should have midwives.

- **The 'good practice' norm** It is important to relate norms based on good practice to their date of origin. A norm may be good practice now, but will it be equally relevant in the future? Managers using this norm will need to build in an element for future improvement in the average staffing levels (upwards or downwards). In other words, they need to make provision for the fact that the basis for the norm may be changing.
- **The 'If ..., then ...' norm** This type of norm is closely related to the good practice norm, but is usually built up by a more objective assessment of staffing requirements in relation to the service provided and tends to be more complex. Many such norms are derived from management service studies. They are based on this type of calculation: if the workload is x and staff can handle y processes per day, then there should be z staff. For example, if 50 immunizations and 50 DOTS treatments are provided per day and one nurse can handle 25 immunizations or 50 DOTS treatments per day, then three nurses are needed.

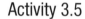

Activity 3.5

List some constraints to the use of norms as a basis for planning a workforce.

Comment

You have probably realized that, in a service as complex as a health system, it is unwise to take any specific staffing norm and apply it throughout the system. The following factors may significantly affect the relevance of any one norm.

- The type of population served by the health system. Is it, for example, predominantly old, rural, well-educated?
- The type of buildings in which the service is provided. Are they new, scattered or previously used for another purpose, such as a church or school?
- The numbers and types of support staff available.
- The source of the norm. Has it been adequately researched or developed by a professional organization primarily interested in expanding its services?

Did you think of any others?

Workload indicators of staffing need (WISN) recognize that staffing requirements vary among health facilities of the same type, based on the consideration of workloads. The need for a workforce based on population ratios or standard staffing schedules is a crude approximation that leads to overstaffing in some facilities (meaning that workers are not fully employed) and understaffing in others (so workers find there is more to do than they can accomplish in working hours). Those facilities that are unable to cope with their workloads underperform – quality and safety of care may be jeopardized and staff suffer stress and low morale.

The WISN method enables health managers to work out the optimal allocation and use of current staff geographically, functionally, by staff categories and their activities. It provides useful information to health administrators at all levels of the health service in times of economic severity and workforce shortages.

POLICIES TO IMPROVE ACCESS TO HEALTHCARE

Policies are needed to improve staff recruitment, deployment, retention and development, as well as more generic policies regarding the conditions of employment and accreditation. This starts with the selection of candidates for training. As discussed earlier, data from a multicountry cross-sectional survey indicated that a substantial proportion of healthcare students planned to move abroad or to urban areas on graduation, although those who came from rural areas and planned at the outset to return to their communities to serve them generally held fast to that ambition.

What is the evidence?

Targeted admissions of rural applicants has been a key component of comprehensive education reforms in developed countries, where schools instituting such policies have increased rural retention from 3–9% to 53–64% of graduates. ... Our data suggest that altering admissions policies in LMIC to favour rural-origin applicants or those desiring to stay in the country will help governments to succeed in retaining health professionals where they are most needed, and to avoid spending public and donor resources on training physicians and nurses most likely to leave.

(Silvestri et al., 2014: 756)

Two commonly used models to develop strategies or policies to improve access to healthcare are the 'working lifespan' and the human resources for health (HRH) action framework.

The World Health Report (2006) proposed the 'working lifespan' approach to systematically address the dynamics of the health workforce by focusing on strategies related to the stage when people enter the workforce, the period of their lives when they are part of the workforce and the point at which they make their exit from it. At each stage, specific policy interventions can be designed and implemented, starting with the development of a national health workforce development plan and continuing with the regulatory frameworks for education and practice (see Figure 3.1).

The HRH action framework is designed to assist governments and health managers when developing and implementing strategies to achieve an effective and sustainable health workforce. By using a comprehensive approach, the framework helps to address staff shortages, uneven distribution of staff, gaps in skills and competences, low retention and poor motivation, among other challenges (Figure 3.2).

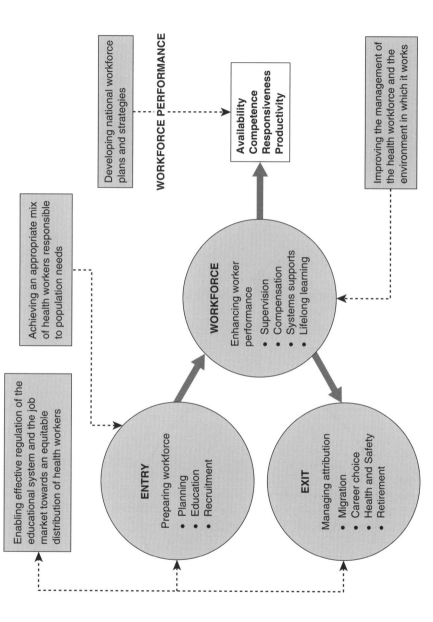

Figure 3.1　Stages of health workforce development

Source: World Health Organization (2006)

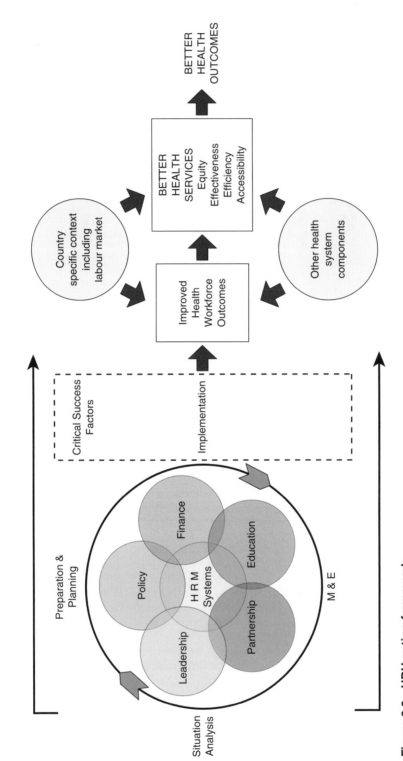

Figure 3.2 HRH action framework

Source: World Health Organization (2008)

CONCLUSION

By 2035, a global deficit of 12.9 million skilled health workers (professionally trained nurses, doctors and midwives) is predicted and this is a major issue when access to universal healthcare of high quality requires innovative solutions delivered by trained staff. Migration, population growth and technological developments also change health needs, so existing staff need to update their skills. While CHWs can be taught to provide health education and basic interventions, supervision and support from clinically trained staff is needed.

Many different occupations need to be planned for, managed and motivated in a functioning health system using SWAps and forecasting to estimate future labour availability and needs. WISN recognizes that staffing requirements vary among health facilities of the same type, based on the consideration of workloads. The need for a workforce based on population ratios or standard staffing schedules is a crude approximation that is widely used.

REFERENCES

Berkley, S., Chan, M., Dybul, M., Hansen, K., Lake, A., Osotimehin, B. and Sidibé, M. (2013) 'A healthy perspective: the post-2015 development agenda', *The Lancet* 381: 1076–77.

Berhan, Y. (2008) 'Medical doctors profile in Ethiopia: production, attrition and retention. In memory of 100-years Ethiopian modern medicine & the new Ethiopian millennium', *Ethiopian Medical Journal*, 46 (S1): 1–77. Available at: www.ncbi.nlm.nih.gov/pubmed/18709707 (accessed 8 October 2015).

Buchan, J., Connell, J. and Rumsey, M. (2011) *Recruiting and Retaining Health Workers in Remote Areas: Pacific Island Case Studies*. Geneva: WHO. Available at: http://whqlibdoc.who.int/publications/2011/9789241501255_eng.pdf?ua=1 (accessed 8 October 2015).

Campbell, J., Buchan, J., Cometto, G., David, B., Dussault, G., Fogstad, H. et al. (2013) 'Human resources for health and universal health coverage: fostering equity and effective coverage', *Bulletin of the World Health Organization*, 91: 853–863. Available at: www.who.int/bulletin/volumes/91/11/13-118729/en/ (accessed 8 October 2015).

HIFA2015 (2014) *Ebola: We Need Health Personnel*. Available at: HIFA205@dgroups.org (accessed 13 October 2015).

McKimm, J., Newton, P.M., Da Silva, A., Campbell, J., Condon, R., Kafoa, B. et al. (2013) *Expanded and Extended Health Practitioner Roles: A Review of International Practice*. Sydney, Australia: Human Resources for Health Knowledge Hub. Available at: http://integrare.es/wp-content/uploads/2014/05/47_SI_Prac-roles_Final.pdf (accessed 8 October 2015).

McPake, B., Maeda, A., Correia Araújo, E., Lemiere, C., El Maghraby, A. and Cometto, G. (2013) 'Why do health labour market forces matter?', *Bulletin of the World Health Organization*, 91: 841–846.

Silvestri, D., Blevins, M. et al. (2014) 'Medical and nursing students' intentions to work abroad or in rural areas: a cross-sectional survey in Asia and Africa', *Bulletin of the World Health Organization*, 92 (10): 750–759.

Task Team for the Global Thematic Consultation on Health in the Post-2015 Development Agenda (2013) 'What do people want for health in the post-2015 agenda?', *The Lancet* 381: 1441–1443.

United Nations General Assembly (2012) *Resolution on Global Health and Foreign Policy*. Available at: www.un.org/ga/search/view_doc.asp?symbol=A/67/L.36 (accessed 8 October 2015).

Vega, J. (2013) 'Universal health coverage: the post-2015 development agenda', *The Lancet*, 381: 179–180.

World Health Organization (n.d.) *Achieving the Health-related MDGs: It Takes a Workforce!* Available at: www.who.int/hrh/workforce_mdgs/en/ (accessed 8 October 2015).

World Health Organization (2006) *Working Together for Health*. The World Health Report. Available at: www.who.int/whr/2006/en/index.html (accessed 8 October 2015).

WHO Regional Office for the Western Pacific (2007) *Regional Strategy on Human Resources for Health 2006–2015*. Manila: World Health Organization.

World Health Organization (2008) *Critical Success. Factors. HRH Action Framework*. Geneva: WHO. Available at: www.who.int/hrh/tools/hrh_action_framework.pdf (accessed 1 October 2015).

WHO (2010) 63rd World Health Assembly. Agenda item 11·5. WHO Global Code of Practice on the International Recruitment of Health Personnel. Available at: http://apps. who.int/gb/ebwha/pdf_files/WHA63/A63_R16-en.pdf (accessed 8 October 2015).

World Health Organization /Global Workforce Alliance (2014) *Human Resources for Health: Foundation for Universal Health Coverage and the Post-2015 Development Agenda: Report of the Third Global Forum on Human Resources for Health*, 10–13 November 2013, Recife, Brazil. Available at: www.who.int/workforcealliance/about/Ag4_3rd_GF_HRH_Report.pdf (accessed 8 October 2015).

PART II
GLOBAL HEALTH IN CONTEXT

HEALTH INEQUALITIES

PHILIPPA K. BIRD AND KATE E. PICKETT

> ### Chapter overview
>
> After reading this chapter you will be able to:
>
> - describe the types and scale of global health inequalities
> - explain the key causes of health inequalities
> - identify implications of the above for practice.

This chapter provides an introduction to socio-economic inequalities in health, both between and within countries, their causes and the implications for policy and practice. Examples are drawn from around the world, with a particular illustration of the contrasting lives led by people born, growing up and living in Nigeria and the countries of the United Kingdom.

HEALTH INEQUALITIES: THE CURRENT SITUATION

A girl born in the United Kingdom is expected to live to 81 years of age. In contrast, a girl born in Nigeria will live to only 54 years, on average (WHO, 2014). There are clearly stark differences in people's health and well-being between countries. Life expectancy now ranges from below 50 years in many sub-Saharan African countries to over 82 years in some European and Western Pacific countries (see Figure 4.1).

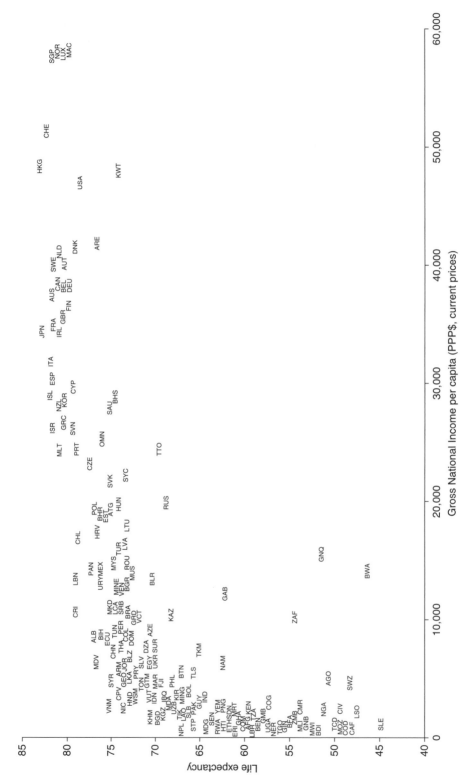

Figure 4.1   Relationship between income per person and life expectancy in rich and poor countries in 2010

Source: World Bank (2010)

Activity 4.1

Figure 4.1 shows the relationship between national income per person and life expectancy in countries worldwide.

Find the following countries on the graph: Botswana (BWA), Vietnam (VNM), and the USA. How does life expectancy in each of these countries compare with other countries that have similar levels of national income per person? Why do you think these differences between countries exist?

Comment

Botswana and the USA have a lower life expectancy than other countries at their respective levels of national income per capita, while the opposite is true for Vietnam. There are many reasons for these differences, including the HIV/AIDS epidemic, levels of social inequality and poverty and the education and health systems in those countries.

These figures conceal inequalities within countries. Children born into the least advantaged households have worse health than those born into more advantaged circumstances. In the UK, children living in less affluent households are more likely to have low birthweight, be shorter and to be in poor health than children in more advantaged households. These inequalities lead to large differences in the number of years that people can expect to live without disability. A woman living in the least deprived areas in England can expect to live to 85 years (of which 70 are disability-free), compared with 80 years (of which 57 are disability-free) for women living in the most deprived areas (ONS, 2013).

Similar patterns are evident in LMICs. The life chances of a child born in Nigeria are strongly shaped by his or her socio-economic circumstances. In 2008, children from the poorest 20 per cent of families in Nigeria were more than twice as likely to die before age five (217 per 1000 live births) than were children from the wealthiest 20 per cent of households (88 per 1000 live births; WHO, 2014).

The effects of social and economic circumstances on health are not confined to those living in poverty. Rather, every incremental increase in socio-economic position confers health and well-being advantages (Adler et al., 1994). This 'social gradient' in health and well-being is evident in both high- and low-income countries. For babies born in England and Wales, there is a finely graded relationship between the level of deprivation in the area in which they live and the chance of infants dying before the age of one. In Nigeria, there is a very high rate of infant mortality, which also has a social gradient. The poorer the child's household, the more likely he or she is to die before the age of one, with babies in the poorest 40 per cent of households being at the greatest risk. Figure 4.2 shows the scale of inequalities in infant mortality, both between and within Nigeria and England and Wales.

Inequalities in health and well-being are also evident by rural/urban residence, ethnicity, gender, educational level and occupation/social class. People who are most vulnerable, disadvantaged and discriminated against experience the worst health and well-being.

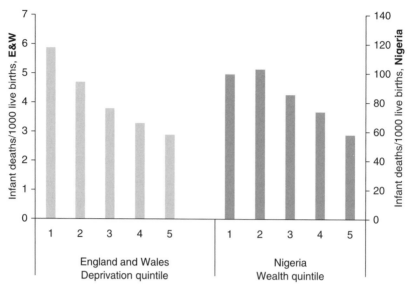

Figure 4.2 **The social gradient in infant mortality in England and Wales and Nigeria**

Source: For England and Wales, infant mortality by quintiles of area deprivation (Carstairs Index), 2005–2006. Redrawn using data from Oakley et al. (2009). For Nigeria, infant mortality by quintiles of household wealth, 2008 (WHO, 2008).

WHY IS THERE A SOCIAL GRADIENT IN HEALTH?

The social and economic conditions that people are born into, grow up and live in shape their health and well-being throughout their lives. In order to understand how these issues influence health, it is useful to think of overlapping influences on health. Individuals have particular characteristics, such as age, sex and lifestyles, that may affect their health. The communities and neighbourhoods that people live in, their working conditions, education, housing quality and other factors affect their health and behaviours. Wider social or economic issues, such as national wealth, income inequality and cultural differences are also important determinants of health.

In order to understand how these social and economic conditions shape people's health, we need to consider the pathways and mechanisms involved. Mechanisms that have been proposed include material resources and living conditions, access to services and infrastructure, the psychological effects of status in society, and differences in health or risky behaviours, such as smoking. The relative importance of each of these may vary between countries and for different health issues. The roles of these pathways may also vary at different points in people's lives.

ABSOLUTE POVERTY AND MATERIAL RESOURCES

It has been recognized for a long time that people with inadequate financial resources and living conditions have poorer health. Public health infrastructure, such as sanitation, as well as improved material living conditions, played a key role in the decline of mortality in Britain in the nineteenth century. Today, however, many people living in absolute poverty continue to lack the material means necessary to achieve good health. People living in poor, overcrowded housing, exposed to air pollution and without clean water and sanitation, are more likely to suffer diseases. People living in poverty may not be able to buy adequate, nutritious food and may also have less resistance to disease because of undernutrition. For example, in Nigeria in 2011, almost two thirds of the population lived below the international poverty line of $1.25 and, in 2012, over one third of people did not have access to clean water and over two thirds did not have access to adequate sanitation facilities (WHO, 2014).

In wealthier countries, few people experience the level of abject poverty experienced in Nigeria. During the economic crisis, the number of people who cannot afford necessities has grown, with large increases in people relying on food banks, but the majority of people have adequate housing and food and the social gradient in health exists even among people who do not live in absolute poverty. This suggests that material living conditions alone cannot explain the gradient in health.

Activity 4.2

List some ways in which the amount of money a person has could affect their health. What goods and services do you need to be able to buy in order to live a healthy life?

Comment

You may have considered items that cost money, such as food, medications, shelter or communications, and the costs of accessing services, such as healthcare, or leisure facilities (including transport costs). Think about what is needed for both mental and physical health. How might this list differ for the UK and Nigeria?

DIFFERENCES IN ACCESS TO SERVICES

Differences in access to services, as well as the quality of the services provided, can be an important cause of inequalities in health within countries. Health facilities and staff are often concentrated in urban and wealthier areas and the costs of services or transportation may prevent people from accessing the care they need. In Nigeria in 2008, only 8 per cent of women from the poorest fifth of households gave birth with the help of a skilled health professional; 86 per cent of women from the wealthiest fifth of households did so (WHO, 2014). People also need to be able to access a range of other services that affect health, such as environmental or social services and, critically, education.

Although many countries have achieved universal coverage of health services, they still have social gradients in health. Inequalities in infant mortality persist in the UK, despite the universal National Health Service. Differences in access and quality of services are unlikely, on their own, to explain the gradient in health.

SOCIAL STATUS AND PSYCHOSOCIAL CAUSES

In the 1970s, the first of several studies of health among civil servants in London – the Whitehall studies – observed that there was a gradient in coronary heart disease by employment grade (Marmot et al., 1978). Indeed, employment grade explained more of the differences in health than conventional risk factors, such as smoking. Yet, civil servants do not lack the material means necessary for health, nor are they exposed to physical occupational hazards. This research led to suggestions that people's position in the social hierarchy relative to others, rather than in absolute terms, is an important cause of health inequalities. In high-income countries (HICs), people may be relatively wealthy in absolute terms by global standards, yet have a low status (in terms of income, education, occupation or other markers of status) relative to others in their society.

There is increasing understanding of psychosocial causes of ill health. Having a low social status relative to others can affect mental and physical health through psychological pathways, including stress, anxiety and social isolation. Living in an unsafe neighbourhood, having job insecurity or financial concerns can be stressful. The work environment is also very important, and feeling a lack of control or reward at work may lead to long-term stress. Chronic stress and anxiety can cause changes in the body's hormonal and nervous systems, which, over time, can have harmful effects on mental health, cardiovascular health and the immune system (Brunner and Marmot, 2006).

Finally, the important role of mental health needs to be recognized. Mental ill health has a steep social gradient and is both disabling in itself and can have detrimental effects on people's health behaviours and physical health. For example, people coping with depression may find it more difficult than those who aren't to engage in healthy behaviours, such as exercise.

HEALTHY AND RISKY BEHAVIOURS

Many healthy and risky behaviours are socially graded. In the UK, there is a clear relationship between socio-economic status and cigarette smoking (Graham et al., 2006). Although many health behaviours are important factors in health inequality, they can only explain a proportion of the social gradient in health in HICs. Dowd (2007) found that maternal behaviours, including smoking, breastfeeding and vitamin use, did not explain the relationship between socio-economic position and child health. Behavioural models are also limited in aiding our understanding of the underlying reasons for people's behaviour – why do people behave as they do? In order to understand this, we also need to consider the roles that material and psychosocial issues play in shaping people's behaviour.

THE IMPORTANCE OF THE LIFE COURSE

Finally, it is important to recognize that health is shaped not only by current circumstances, but also by the long-term effects of circumstances earlier in the life course. Being exposed to adverse circumstances during critical or particularly sensitive periods of growth or development may lead to disease later in life. Poor foetal growth in utero (marked by low birthweight) has been shown to be associated with coronary heart disease (CHD), stroke, diabetes and respiratory disease in adulthood (Barker, 1998). Risks or damage can also accumulate over the life course. A study of the association between childhood socio-economic status and CHD in adult men found that men who experienced low socio-economic positions in both childhood and adulthood had the highest risk of CHD, illustrating how damage from low socio-economic status accumulated during the life course (Ramsay et al., 2007).

Children growing up in disadvantaged circumstances may be exposed to a range of biological behavioural material and psychosocial risk factors, with long-term adverse effects on their health and development. This begins in utero, when maternal nutrition and low levels of stress are essential for healthy foetal development. If mothers are stressed during pregnancy, their adult children are likely to have cognitive or emotional problems (Talge et al., 2007). After birth, children's experiences in the first few years of life affect their health as adults. These first years are a critical period for brain development. A recent review of the risk factors for early child development in LMICs identified biological factors, such as iodine or iron deficiency, HIV infection and malaria, and psychosocial factors, such as maternal depression and inadequate cognitive stimulation, as particularly detrimental for early brain development (Walker et al., 2011).

DIRECTION OF CAUSALITY AND SOCIAL SELECTION

Health or illness could act as a selecting force that pushes people into better or worse socio-economic circumstances. This 'social selection' model suggests that a person's position in society results from his or her level of 'fitness' or health. So, a child with chronic illness might achieve a low level of education and, in turn, obtain a low-paid job; conversely, someone who is healthy might perform well in education and work and obtain a higher-status profession and income.

There is evidence that illness and the costs of healthcare can push people into poverty in LMICs where access to care and social support are limited – the 'medical poverty trap' (Whitehead et al., 2001). Even in HICs, with universal healthcare and welfare systems, severe illness can cause financial strain and impoverishment. A study of the costs of cancer among young people highlighted the economic strain on households arising from treatment costs coupled with the loss of income when parents took time off work to care for their children. As a result, two thirds of parents and half of young people had to borrow money to make ends meet (CLIC Sargent, 2011).

The evidence for social selection, however, is mixed and varies by country and health problem. Socio-economic disadvantage usually occurs before poor health and selection alone cannot explain the extent of the social gradient in health (Adler et al., 1994).

─────────────────────── Activity 4.3 ───────────────────────

There are clear social gradients in child nutrition in Nigeria and in England. In Nigeria, the poorer the household that children live in, the higher the probability that they are malnourished. It was found in 2011 that 10 per cent of children under five in the richest fifth of households were underweight for their age, while 38 per cent were in the poorest fifth of households (UNICEF, 2014).

(Continued)

(Continued)

In England, relatively few children are underweight and there is not a marked social gradient. Child obesity, however, is a growing problem and has a steep social gradient. In 2013–2014, 7 per cent of children aged four to five in the least deprived tenth of areas were obese, while 12 per cent of children living in the most deprived tenth of areas were obese (HSCIC, 2014).

For each of the following questions, consider the role of material factors, services and policies, psychosocial factors and behavioural factors. Think about the similarities and differences between the two countries.

1. Why are children living in the most disadvantaged circumstances in Nigeria more likely to be underweight than those in less disadvantaged circumstances?
2. Why are children living in the most disadvantaged circumstances in England more likely to be overweight than those in the least deprived areas?
3. What would be the best strategies to reduce the inequalities in nutrition in the two countries?

Comment

This activity encourages you to consider the role of the setting in which the disadvantage occurs and how it may have different implications for health. You could have considered the implications of having insufficient money in terms of the types or quantity of food that you can buy in each country. You could also have considered the role of factors such as time and knowledge to prepare healthy meals or how living in a deprived area might affect the amount of activity that children participate in. In addition, you could also have considered the growing number of countries that have problems with both obesity and undernutrition, such as Brazil or India.

WHY ARE THERE INEQUALITIES IN HEALTH BETWEEN COUNTRIES?

The explanations for the differences in health between countries have considerable overlap with the causes of the social gradient in health within countries. For LMICs, the level of national wealth is critical for health. Figure 4.1 showed the relationship between national income per person and life expectancy in 2010. For the poorest countries (under $10,000 per person), there was a very steep relationship between income and life expectancy. For countries earning above $10,000 per person, this relationship was less steep. Once countries achieved over $25,000 per person, the relationship between wealth and health was flat – that is, for wealthier countries, gains in national income did not bring about better health.

For LMICs, a higher national income would enable greater spending on essential services for health, especially education and health services, and better welfare and support. At the household level, higher income facilitates spending on the resources and services needed for health. Higher levels of national income do not always lead to better health, however, as political factors come into play. If increases in income and improvements in services are distributed inequitably, the benefits may be confined to those in more advantaged circumstances. In Figure 4.1 we saw that there is considerable variation in the levels of health achieved by countries at the same level of income. Sri Lanka, for example, was poorer than Pakistan, but had achieved a life expectancy over seven years longer than Pakistan. This may reflect Sri Lanka's emphasis on equity and government investment in education and health services.

In HICs, the distribution of income among the population (income inequality) is a more important predictor of health than the level of national wealth. Studies have shown the importance of income inequality for a wide range of health and social outcomes, including adult and infant mortality, life expectancy, self-rated health and violent crime (Wilkinson and Pickett, 2009a). Figure 4.3 shows how infant mortality rates are closely related to the level of income inequality. Countries with the most equal distribution of income, such as Japan and Finland, have very low levels of infant mortality. In contrast, the most unequal countries, such as the USA and UK, have high levels of infant mortality.

A number of explanations for this relationship between income inequality and health have been put forward. These also reflect the causes of the social gradient, discussed earlier. Some have suggested that income inequality affects health as a result of material factors, as well as the level of investment in infrastructure and services (Lynch et al., 2000). These factors may affect health behaviours or health directly. More equal countries also tend to have more progressive policies and equitable access to services, benefiting health and well-being. This explanation suggests that the health effects of inequality are not inevitable and could be reduced through more equitable public policies and services.

Living in a society with high levels of inequality also has a range of psychosocial effects on individuals and communities, including increased status differentiation

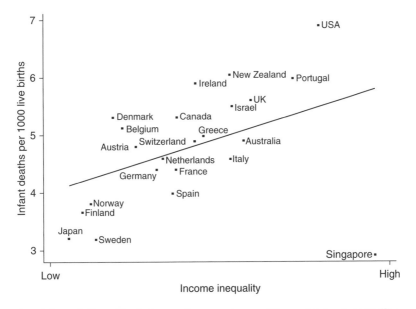

Figure 4.3 The relationship between income inequality and infant mortality

Source: Wilkinson and Pickett (2009b)

and lower social cohesion. In highly unequal societies, with high levels of status differentiation, people compare themselves with others in their society, which can lead to stress and negative emotions. This has a negative impact on health directly and indirectly by influencing health behaviours. Social cohesion also tends to be lower in more unequal societies, with people in such countries less likely to trust others, which has implications for mental and physical health (Wilkinson and Pickett, 2009a).

The suggestion that health tends to be better in more equal countries was first put forward over 25 years ago. Since then, over 300 studies have analyzed the link between income inequality and a wide range of health and social outcomes. The relationship between income inequality and health is very difficult to study, however, and there are some inconsistencies between studies. There are several reasons for these different findings.

First, the health outcomes that are most closely related to income inequality are the outcomes with a steep social gradient, such as infant mortality or mental illness (Wilkinson and Pickett, 2009a). Second, income inequality at the national level (or state level in the USA) is often related to population health, but there is less evidence from studies that have looked at income inequality in small areas. There may also be a time lag between changes in income inequality and changes in health. A more recent review concluded that the evidence meets established epidemiological and other scientific criteria for causality (Pickett and Wilkinson, 2015).

WHAT CAN BE DONE TO REDUCE INEQUALITIES IN HEALTH?

In order to reduce inequalities in health, policies and interventions need to tackle the root causes. This requires a focus on the overlapping social determinants of health, mechanisms and pathways to health inequalities.

TACKLING THE ROOT CAUSES OF HEALTH INEQUALITY

In order to tackle the root causes of health inequality, structural changes to the unequal distribution of social and economic resources are required. This applies both to global inequities between countries and social and economic inequality within countries. Since 1980, a number of high-profile reports on health inequalities have been published in the UK and with an international focus (Acheson, 1998; Black, 1980; Commission on Social Determinants of Health, 2008; Marmot, 2010). These reports produced recommendations stressing the need to address the social determinants of health and all emphasized the need to address economic inequality.

This priority is shared by public health researchers. In a recent survey of support for different policy options to tackle health inequalities, there was support for more progressive distribution of income and wealth and greater investment in public services in deprived communities (Smith and Eltanani, 2014). The current evidence base is stronger for interventions with a behavioural or health systems focus and there is a need for more clear evidence on interventions to tackle the social determinants of health.

What is the evidence?

The Commission on Social Determinants of Health

The Commission on Social Determinants of Health compiled the evidence for what can be done to promote health equity at a global level (Commission on Social Determinants of Health, 2008). Their report focused on inequalities both between and within countries at different levels of wealth and development. The authors identified a range of recommendations to reduce inequalities in health, with the following three overarching recommendations.

1. **Improve daily living conditions** The social determinants of health should be tackled by improving daily living conditions. This includes an emphasis on early child development and education. The Commission also called for policies to improve living and working conditions throughout adult life and into older life.
2. **Tackle the inequitable distribution of power, money, and resources** Tackle inequalities in the way the society is organized – that is, the structural drivers of people's daily living conditions. The report called for strengthened and fair financing of action on the social determinants of health and noted the need for a strong public sector with strengthened governance.
3. **Measure and understand the problem and assess the impact of action** Acknowledge and measure the problem of health inequity (both within and between countries). They called for routine monitoring of health inequity and the social determinants of health, as well as evaluation of the impact of policies and action on health equity.

Before we move on to the next section – and to consolidate your understanding of how health equity can be promoted by health professionals – complete the following activity.

───────────────── Activity 4.4 ─────────────────

Read the summary above of the Commission on Social Determinants of Health's overarching recommendations. You can access the full report or executive summary online at: www.who.int/social_determinants/thecommission/finalreport

What role can health professionals play in actioning each of the three overarching recommendations? Consider what health professionals can do to a) implement and b) advocate for these policies and interventions.

Comment

Were you surprised by the number of languages in which this report is available? Were you put off by the length of the report?

You could have thought of actions that you have seen health professionals taking in the past or you could develop new, innovative ideas for action.

THE ROLE OF HEALTH PROFESSIONALS

The root causes of ill health (such as lack of education, poor income and working conditions) lie outside the traditional focus of the clinical health system, although they have always been a focus for public health professionals. In order to tackle health inequality, therefore, health professionals need to focus on wider determinants of health, as well as on improvements within the health system. Inequalities in access to healthcare and the costs of illness remain, even in universal health systems. Health professionals, policymakers and implementers in the health system therefore have an important role to play in ensuring fair access to high-quality healthcare and that the costs of ill health and treatment do not push households into poverty.

Evidence and recommendations for how health professionals can expand their work to focus on the social determinants of health are provided in a recent overview of health professionals' roles (Allen et al., 2013). Partnership work with professionals in other sectors, such as education services or charities, and referral of patients to non-medical services enable health professionals to play a greater role in disease prevention. Scope for this is often limited in secondary healthcare, but there is greater opportunity within primary healthcare, and intersectoral work is a focus in public health organizations. A range of initiatives have been trialled in the UK, including assessment of housing needs for elderly patients during health contacts and the co-location of services within GP clinics, in order to help address the social and economic environments that patients live in (Allen et al., 2013).

Perhaps most importantly, health professionals and professional bodies have a key advocacy role to improve the social and economic conditions that shape people's lives. Advocacy work could include support for local and national policies that tackle the root causes of inequalities, as well as opposition to policies that may be harmful to people's health. Health professionals are in a position of authority to highlight the causes of health inequality, advocate the fairer distribution of resources in society and promote greater health equality.

──────────────────────────── Activity 4.5 ────────────────────────────

This chapter has highlighted some of the inequalities between and within countries worldwide. As you read the other chapters in this book, try to be aware of these inequalities. Consider whether or not there are differences in people's experiences, either between or within countries. Thinking about health using an 'equity lens' will help you to identify inequalities, their causes and possible ways to reduce them and their impacts.

Comment

Remember to think about inequalities in the range of factors related to people's health, such as their health outcomes, the distribution and quality of health services, health behaviours, stress and mental health, the financial effects of suffering poor health, housing conditions and work environment, among others.

CONCLUSION

This chapter has provided an overview of health inequalities, both between and within countries, the causes of these inequalities and the role that health professionals can play. There are vast inequalities in health between countries, and between people living in different socio-economic circumstances within countries. These have been illustrated by the differences in health between people living in Nigeria and the United Kingdom and the social gradient in health in both countries. Causes of the social gradient in health within countries include poverty and material resources, access to health services, social status and psychosocial causes, healthy and risky behaviours and their influences throughout the life course. Comparing countries with different levels of income, life expectancy is related to national income per capita among LMICs, but, among HICs, health is more closely related to the distribution of income. Policies and service provision, such as education, health services and welfare systems, also play an important role. Health professionals can also play a role in the identification of health inequalities and actions to improve equality, including ensuring the equitable provision of health services, working with other sectors to improve health and advocating the promotion of health equality.

REFERENCES

Acheson, D. (1998) *Independent Inquiry into Inequalities in Health*. London: The Stationery Office.

Adler, N.E., Boyce, T., Chesney, M.A., Cohen, S., Folkman, S., Kahn, R.L. et al. (1994) 'Socioeconomic status and health. The challenge of the gradient', *Am Psychol*, 49: 15–24.

Allen, M., Allen, J., Hogarth, S. and Marmot, M. (2013) *Working for Health Equity: The Role of Health Professionals*. London: UCL Institute of Health Equity.

Barker D. (1998) *Mothers, Babies and Health in Later Life*. Edinburgh: Churchill Livingstone.

Black, D. (1980) *Inequalities in Health: Report of a Research Working Group*. London: Penguin.

Brunner, E. and Marmot, M. (2006) 'Social organization, stress, and health'. In M. Marmot and R.G. Wilkinson (eds) *Social Determinants of Health*, 2nd edition. Oxford: Oxford University Press, pp. 6–30.

CLIC Sargent (2011) *Counting the Costs of Cancer. The Financial Impact of Cancer on Children, Young People and their Families*. London: CLIC Sargent. Available at: www.clicsargent.org.uk/sites/files/clicsargent/Countingthecostsofcancerreport.pdf (accessed 8 October 2015).

Commission on Social Determinants of Health (2008) *Closing the Gap in a Generation: Health Equity through Action on the Social Determinants of Health. Final Report of the Commission on Social Determinants of Health*. Geneva: World Health Organization.

Dowd, J.B. (2007) 'Early childhood origins of the income/health gradient: the role of maternal health behaviors', *Social Science & Medicine*, 65: 1202–1213.

Graham, H., Inskip, H.M., Francis, B. and Harman, J. (2006) 'Pathways of disadvantage and smoking careers: evidence and policy implications', *Journal of Epidemiology and Community Health*, 60: ii7–ii12.

HSCIC (2014) *National Child Measurement Programme: England, 2013/14 School Year*. Health and Social Care Information Centre.

Lynch, J.W., Davey Smith, G., Kaplan, G.A. and House, J.S. (2000) 'Income inequality and mortality: importance to health of individual income, psychosocial environment, or material conditions', *British Medical Journal*, 320: 1200–1204.

Marmot, M.G. (2010) *Fair Society, Healthy Lives (The Marmot Review)*. Available at: www.instituteofhealthequity.org/projects/fair-society-healthy-lives-the-marmot-review (accessed 8 October 2015).

Marmot, M.G., Rose, G., Shipley, M. and Hamilton, P.J. (1978) 'Employment grade and coronary heart disease in British civil servants', *Journal of Epidemiology and Community Health*, 32: 244–249.

Oakley, L., Maconochie, N., Doyle, P., Dattani, N. and Moser, K. (2009) 'Multivariate analysis of infant death in England & Wales in 2005/06, with focus on socio-economic status and deprivation', *Health Statistics Quarterly*, 42: 22–39.

ONS (2013) *Inequality in Disability-Free Life Expectancy by Area Deprivation: England, 2003–06 and 2007–10*. London: Office for National Statistics.

Pickett, K.E. and Wilkinson, R.G. (2015) 'Income inequality and health: a causal review', *Social Science & Medicine*. 128 316e326

Ramsay, S.E., Whincup, P.H., Morris, R.W., Lennon, L.T. and Wannamethee, S.G. (2007) 'Are childhood socio-economic circumstances related to coronary heart disease risk? Findings from a population-based study of older men', *International Journal of Epidemiology*, 36: 560–566.

Smith, K.E. and Eltanani, M.K. (2014) 'What kinds of policies to reduce health inequalities in the UK do researchers support?', *Journal of Public Health*, published online 30 August.

Talge, N.M., Neal, C. and Glover, V. (2007) 'Antenatal maternal stress and long-term effects on child neurodevelopment: how and why?', *Journal of Child Psychology and Psychiatry*, 48: 245–261.

UNICEF (2014) *The State of the World's Children 2014: Every Child Counts*. New York: UNICEF.

Walker, S.P., Wachs, T.D., Grantham-McGregor, S., Black, M.M., Nelson, C.A., Huffman, S.L. et al. (2011) 'Inequality in early childhood: risk and protective factors for early child development', *The Lancet*, 378: 1325–1338.

Whitehead, M., Dahlgren, G. and Evans, T. (2001) 'Equity and health sector reforms: can low-income countries escape the medical poverty trap?', *The Lancet*, 358: 833–836.

Wilkinson, R.G. and Pickett, K.E. (2009a) 'Income inequality and social dysfunction', *Annual Review of Sociology*, 35: 493–511.

Wilkinson, R.G. and Pickett, K.E. (2009b) *The Spirit Level: Why Equality is Better for Everyone*. London: Penguin.

WHO (2008) *Demographic and Health Surveys, Health Equity Monitor*. Geneva: WHO.

WHO (2014) *World Health Statistics 2014*. Geneva: WHO.

The World Bank (2010) *World Development Indicators 2010*. Washington, DC: World Bank. Available from: http://data.worldbank.org/data-catalog/world-development-indicators/wdi-2010 (accessed 8 October 2015).

5

HUMAN HEALTH AND THE GLOBAL ENVIRONMENT

STEFI BARNA, JASON HORSLEY AND SARAH WALPOLE

Chapter overview

After reading this chapter you will be able to:

- describe the mechanisms through which human health depends on ecological systems
- recognize the sources, pathways, impacts and control measures for environmentally mediated disease
- discuss the contribution of human activity to global environmental changes – in particular, to climate change
- describe the processes through which climate change exacerbates health inequity.

INTRODUCTION

Over the last two centuries, dramatic improvements in nutrition, sanitation and access to healthcare have allowed humans to live longer, healthier lives. In 1800, the average life expectancy globally was approximately 30 years; two centuries later it was 66 years. Over the same period, global population increased from one to seven billion.

Most advances in population health stem from technological mastery of the relationship between humans and the natural environment. For example, with technology and fossil fuels, we have created an infrastructure to bring clean drinking water to billions of people, designed systems to water, fertilize, harvest and transport the food to nourish them and invented chemical insecticides to reduce transmission of vector-borne diseases.

Technological advances have also created new hazards for human health, however, including chemical pollution, nuclear radiation and climate change. The health burdens of these hazards are distributed unequally between and within populations.

In this chapter, we explore the physical, chemical and biological components of environmental health and the new threat of climate change.

THE ENVIRONMENTAL DETERMINANTS OF HEALTH

Many factors determine whether or not an individual will live a long and healthy life or suffer from early disease, disability or death. These social determinants of health include whether or not our neighbourhoods are safe and healthy, we have access to clean water and air and our societies are supported by well-functioning ecological systems and a stable climate (see Chapter 6).

Children are particularly sensitive to environmental hazards, whether biological (such as microbes), chemical (such as toxins) or physical (such as radiation). The WHO estimates that nearly one third of the 6.6 million deaths of children under the age of five each year are associated with environment-related causes and conditions, including diarrhoeal disease and malaria. The release of tens of thousands of new chemicals since the 1950s coincides with rapidly rising incidences of childhood asthma, obesity, diabetes, attention deficit hyperactivity disorder (ADHD) and birth defects. Protecting children from biological and chemical hazards is

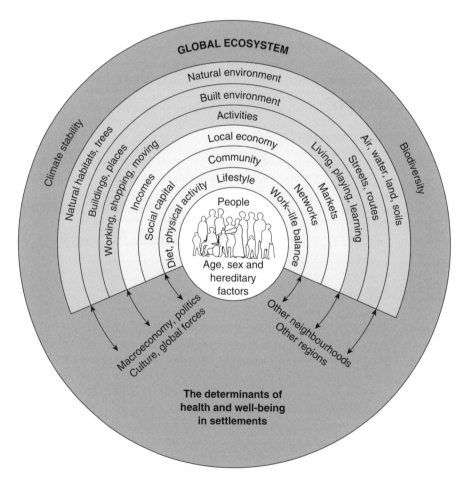

Figure 5.1　Social determinants of health include human-made environmental hazards

Source: Barton and Grant (2006). Reproduced by permission of SAGE Publications Ltd.

technically possible but not always prioritized by government policy and business practices. Figure 5.1 illustrates how social determinants of health are dependent on and influenced by the environmental context.

PLANETARY BOUNDARIES

With a steady input of fluid, food and micronutrients, our bodies can maintain homeostasis and preserve all their vital parameters within the narrow range needed for optimal functioning. When an organ fails or a toxin is introduced, these homeostatic mechanisms become overwhelmed, resulting in rapid accumulation of toxins and a progressive loss of equilibrium.

The Earth also has mechanisms to maintain the equilibrium of its biosphere. Energy (in the form of heat and light) arrives from the sun and drives the water, nitrogen and carbon cycles. Today, there is scientific consensus that our species has altered the biosphere's equilibrium. Figure 5.2 describes the 'planetary boundaries' of essential

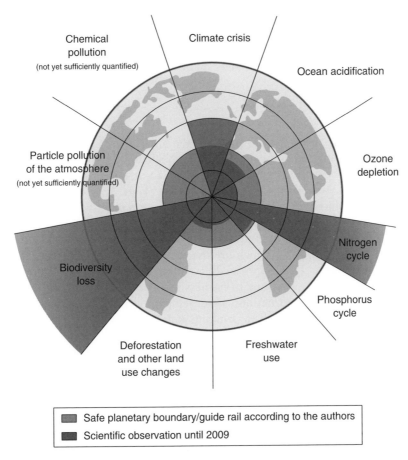

Figure 5.2 Geophysical planetary 'boundaries'

Source: Nature (2009). Reprinted by permission from Macmillan Publishers Ltd.

Earth-system processes and how close we may be to breaching those boundaries. The areas of most concern are climate change, loss of biodiversity and disruption of the nitrogen cycle. In other areas (chemical pollution, land degradation, freshwater use, ocean acidification and ozone depletion) the threshold limits have not yet been quantified (Rocksrom et al., 2009). Breaching the boundaries will undermine the ecosystem processes needed to support our population of seven billion people.

CLIMATE CHANGE

The Earth's climate varies naturally over time. 'Climate' is defined as the average weather over a period of time, usually calculated from the mean and variability of temperature, precipitation and wind over a 30-year period. When we talk about 'climate change', however, we usually mean changes that are anthropogenic – that is, caused by humans – and result in an increase in the average global temperatures above and beyond the normal variations of the Earth's geological history.

Anthropogenic climate change is caused by the accumulation of gases in the atmosphere that prevent the sun's heat from radiating back into space. These gases are called 'greenhouse' gases. Some greenhouse gases (including carbon dioxide, methane, nitrous oxide and ozone) are more effective at warming the Earth than others, and some can remain in the atmosphere for hundreds or thousands of years. In this chapter, we focus on carbon dioxide (CO_2) because it is the primary human-created contributor to global warming.

UNLEASHING STORED ENERGY

The amount of carbon on the Earth and in the atmosphere is fixed and constantly moving between living and non-living things. Through photosynthesis, plants take CO_2 out of the atmosphere and release oxygen. This CO_2 is converted into carbon compounds and stored. Animals absorb carbon by eating plants. Animals breathe in oxygen and exhale CO_2, which is then available for plants to use in photosynthesis. When plants die and decompose, their carbon is released into the atmosphere or stored in the soil.

For much of Earth's history, large amounts of carbon have been locked up in fossil fuels – coal, oil and gas – which are the remnants of organic matter that lived millions of years ago. The Industrial Revolution unlocked the enormous energy stored in fossil fuels. We continue to harness this energy today to improve health, particularly in industrialized nations, by developing infrastructure, goods' production and transport, access to clean drinking water, food, and electricity for homes and workplaces. We also use energy to power transport and machines to make our lives easier, reducing the amount of personal energy we use for work and travel. This 'high-carbon' lifestyle, in which energy from fossil fuels replaces the human energy powered by food, is part of what is called 'development'.

Burning fossil fuels has released carbon compounds into the atmosphere (as CO_2 and other gases) at a much faster rate than they would have been released naturally. Other human processes, such as clearing large areas of forest for agriculture or settlements, has reduced the Earth's capacity to store carbon. We are beginning to recognize the need for a more sustainable model of development, building societies that can meet the needs of the current generation without impairing the capacity of future generations to look after their own needs.

--------------------------------- Activity 5.1 ---------------------------------

All animals, including humans, need access to basic resources such as oxygen, water, food and a habitable climate. When these resources are scarce, we are often willing to fight for them. Although often masked by issues of religion or politics, most wars are the result of groups of people struggling to obtain or maintain access to natural resources such as agricultural land, fresh water, oil, coal and natural gas. The combination of a growing population, rising consumer expectations and an unstable climate is likely to exacerbate the frequency and intensity of conflicts over resources. In addition to civilian deaths and displacement, wars destroy infrastructure that can take decades to replace and population health deteriorates rapidly when food, water and electricity supplies are interrupted.

Make a list of resources that people are willing to fight for. Look up situations in which conflict has occurred over scarcity of resources.

Comment

The Romans fought the Punic Wars (264–146BCE) to gain control of grain production in the fertile valleys of North Africa, Sardinia and Corsica. Hitler justified his 1939 invasion of Poland by saying that it provided 'lebensraum' (living room) for the German people. Saddam Hussein's 1990 invasion of Kuwait was precipitated by a battle over ownership of an oilfield. Russia's 2014 annexation of Crimea may be seen as an attempt to gain control over the 'breadbasket' of the Soviet Union. A chain of remote, energy-rich islands known as Senkaku (in Japan) and Diaoyu (in China) are the subject of an escalating territorial dispute.

IS CLIMATE CHANGE HAPPENING?

The UN's Intergovernmental Panel on Climate Change (IPCC) has been monitoring scientific research on global temperature change since 1988. The 2014 report concludes that the average temperature of the Earth's surface has risen by 0.6°C since the late 1800s and is expected to increase by a minimum of 1.4°C by the year 2100. This increase is larger than any century-long trend in the past 10,000 years and is primarily due to human activity. In a worst-case scenario, it may rise by over 4°C – an increase that would make it difficult for large-scale human civilizations to survive.

HOW DO WE KNOW?

Since the 1950s, scientists have measured increases in concentrations of greenhouse gases in the atmosphere. Temperature data collected from ancient sources (fossil records, pollen counts in ancient bogs, and isotopes of oxygen and hydrogen in ice cores) show a strong correlation between temperature and atmospheric CO_2 over the last 420,000 years and, for the majority of this time, the Earth was much colder, with occasional 'interglacial' periods lasting about 10,000 to 30,000 years. Temperature data from tree rings, ships' logs and meteorological stations show that the planet has warmed about 1°C over the past 150 years. Over the past 50 years, there has been an exponential rise in the concentration of CO_2 in the atmosphere. Current levels of CO_2 exceed any measured even in the oldest ice cores. In short, CO_2 levels are now higher than at any time in the history of human life on the planet.

It is predicted that a rise in global temperature of more than 4°C would have a catastrophic effect on current ecological cycles, partly due to 'tipping points' in the climate system. Normally, equilibrium is maintained by negative feedback cycles, where a shift in one direction (such as an increase in temperature or acidity) triggers mechanisms that oppose the change (reduce temperature or acidity).

A tipping point occurs when a change triggers a positive feedback cycle. A small change in one direction triggers further changes in the same direction. An example of a positive feedback cycle is that increasing global temperatures trigger the melting of permafrost and the release of large amounts of methane stored in tundra. Methane is a greenhouse gas 20 times more potent than CO_2, so its release triggers rapid further warming.

Tipping point scenarios are complex and difficult to predict with mathematical models, hence the critical levels at which they occur are usually unclear. Further examples of climate tipping points include the melting of the Greenland ice sheet, dieback of the Amazon rainforest and the shift of the West African monsoon.

IS IT CAUSED BY HUMAN ACTIVITY?

The term 'anthropogenic climate change' refers to the global warming that is due to human activity. Humans are the major cause of the current level of global warming, due to population growth, urbanization and the demand for transportation, electricity and processed goods. Nearly half a trillion tonnes of carbon-based fossil fuels have been burned to drive our current lifestyles. Coupled with deforestation for agriculture and building, the burning of fossil fuels by humans has transformed planetary ecosystems (see Figure 5.2).

Between 1959 and 2008, about 43 per cent of each year's CO_2 emissions remained in the atmosphere, while 57 per cent was absorbed naturally into land and ocean 'carbon sinks'. The proportion of CO_2 emissions removed from the atmosphere decreased over the period, from about 60 per cent to 55 per cent. Models suggest that this trend was caused by a decrease in the uptake of CO_2 by carbon sinks due to climate change and variability.

Activity 5.2

We are producing CO_2 faster than the Earth can absorb it. We can address this problem by accessing renewable energy sources (such as solar, wind and tidal power), reducing the amount of energy we use (consuming fewer material goods and travelling less, for example) or using energy more efficiently (by insulating houses or growing food closer to where it is consumed, for example). Which of these options do you think should be prioritized? How feasible is each option? What are the practical, social, health and political issues involved?

WHAT CAN BE DONE?

Greenhouse gases that have accumulated in the atmosphere since the Industrial Revolution have already caused the Earth to warm by 0.8°C more than it would have done naturally. Some scientific models suggest that global warming can still be capped at a level that we might be able to manage (2°C), with immediate and substantial reductions in greenhouse gas emissions. Other models predict that keeping the temperature rise below 2°C is unlikely or impossible.

Preparing for the changes that result from global warming is called 'climate change adaptation'. Adaptation measures include building heatwave warning systems and defences to protect land from flooding and rises in the sea level, developing new agricultural crops for altered climates and improving living conditions and livelihood prospects for climate refugees.

In addition to managing changes that we cannot prevent, we must try to prevent climate change we cannot manage: 'climate change mitigation'. International proposals for climate change mitigation include reducing the quantity of fossil fuels burned and protecting forests, which absorb carbon. Mitigation policies can seem expensive until the cost savings of a reduced level of climate change adaptation are included. In addition, many climate impacts – such as the loss of human lives, cultural heritage and damage to ecosystem services – are difficult to value and monetize.

Implementing effective adaptation and mitigation practices requires the involvement of many sectors, including healthcare. Sustainable development addresses the environmental, social and economic dimensions involved in the transition to sustainable societies and communities.

Activity 5.3

National governments have traditionally had three roles: protecting the country from foreign invasion, maintaining order within the country, and raising revenues. Over the last century, their role has expanded to include developing infrastructure, providing social welfare and supporting economic growth. But what is a country's responsibility with regard to global environmental change? The following activity encourages you to think about factors that would influence whether or not national governments support international commitments to prevent climate change.

Make a table with two columns. In the left-hand column, make a list of possible reasons for a government acting to reduce climate change. In the right-hand column make a list of reasons for it perhaps not wanting to act. You may want to find out what actions are being taken by your government currently. You could also consider the differences between democratic and authoritarian forms of government.

Comment

Reasons to take action	Reasons to avoid action
Concern for long-term economic or environmental sustainability of the country.	Fossil fuels cheaply available.
Desire to position country at the forefront of new technologies by subsidizing sustainable energy.	No domestic alternative to fossil fuels or a pre-existing commitment to subsidize fossil fuels.
Response to popular demand.	Response to pressure from corporate interests.

HEALTH AND CLIMATE CHANGE

The current worldwide burden of ill health due to climate change is not well quantified, but conservative estimates suggest that it already causes 200,000 premature deaths each year. Over 85 per cent of climate change-related deaths occur in LICs, predominantly in sub-Saharan Africa and South Asia, and involve children under the age of five. Until the middle of the century, climate change will exacerbate existing health problems and extend the range of vector and water-borne disease into new areas.

Even in HICs, considerable evidence suggests that preparation is needed to minimize climate change-related harms. For example, elevated temperatures in the 2003 European heatwave resulted in over 30,000 heat-related deaths, plus flooding has caused billions of dollars of damage and significant loss of life. Vulnerable populations – children, older people, and those living in poverty, in certain geographic areas or with underlying health conditions – are at even greater risk from climate change having an impact on their health.

Climate change is expected to affect health in three ways (see Table 5.1).

Short-term and direct risks from injury, disease and death occur due to extreme weather events (heatwaves, storms and flooding). Longer-term risks include those posed by changes to air quality, such as increased concentrations of ground-level ozone inflaming people's airways, making acute exacerbation of asthma and emphysema more likely. Air pollution is associated with increased risk of ischaemic stroke and myocardial infarction.

Indirect risks arise from changes and disruptions to ecological and biophysical systems, affecting food yields, the production of aeroallergens (spores and pollens), bacterial growth rates, the range and activity of disease vectors (such as mosquitoes) and water flows and quality. The indirect effects of climate change will cause the greatest number of disability-adjusted life years (DALYs) and deaths, but may be less noticeable because they occur slowly, follow complex causal pathways and occur in poorer countries with less robust recordkeeping.

CLIMATE CHANGE AND HEALTH INEQUITY

The health impacts of climate change and energy use are unevenly distributed. Disadvantaged communities are not only the most likely to be exposed to climate-related health threats but also more likely to become unwell as a result (they have a higher level of vulnerability) and have the fewest resources to respond to illness. The risk of weather-related natural disasters is almost 80 times higher in LICs than it is in HICs. More than half of urban dwellers in Africa and Asia lack access to adequate water and sanitation and one billion people in LICs live in slums. Meanwhile, HICs have used fossil fuel energy to improve nutrition and sanitation, build up infrastructure and combat infectious diseases. Within countries, it is the poorer members of society who are more likely to lack access to clean water, sanitation and healthcare; more likely to experience adverse working conditions during periods of excess urban heat; and more likely to go hungry when food prices rise due to climate change.

The poorest one billion people in the world produce only 3 per cent of global anthropogenic carbon emissions. The illness burden therefore overwhelmingly falls on those who have contributed least to the problem of climate change.

Table 5.1 Pathways by which climate change affects health

Category	Mechanism	Mediator of health impact	Examples
1. Short Term Direct Risks	Heatwaves	Heat stress and dehydration make deaths from heatstroke, stroke, cardiac disease, respiratory conditions and diabetes more likely. Risk is highest in children, the aged and manual workers.	Europe's month-long heatwave in 2003 resulted in at least 35,000 excess deaths (compared to years without heatwaves). In the USA, every 1 degree increment in average temperatures increases the risk of basal cell carcinoma by 2.9 per cent and squamous cell carcinoma by 5.5 per cent.
	More frequent extreme weather events (floods, storms)	Compromised water sanitation (due to damage to water systems and run-off from farms) causes increases in infectious diseases, such as malaria, cholera and other gastrointestinal infections.	Severe flooding in Dhaka, Bangladesh, in 1998 was associated with an increase in diarrhoea during and afterwards.
2. Longer Term Direct Risks	Air quality	Greenhouse gases, such as ozone, and the airborne pollutants associated with fossil fuel combustion contribute to an array of respiratory and cardiovascular disease through inflammation of the airways.	Greenhouse gas emissions are responsible for an estimated 1.3 million deaths a year.
		Airborne ash from drought-related wildfires contributes to a rise in asthma.	Australian studies suggest that, for every $10\mu g/m^3$ increase in the daily average concentration of fine particulate matter, health-impaired populations risk a 4 per cent increase in mortality.
		Higher levels of atmospheric CO_2 act as a fertilizer for plant growth. Temperature changes are expected to initiate earlier and longer-lasting allergy seasons and a change in the distribution of allergenic plant varieties.	In the eastern USA, a doubling of atmospheric CO_2 has caused a tripling of pollen production.

(Continued)

Table 5.1 (Continued)

Category	Mechanism	Mediator of health impact	Examples
3. Indirect Risks	Reductions in food yield	A rise in sea level and changes in rainfall patterns reduce crop yields and increase prices. Malnutrition increases susceptibility to infectious disease, stunting of growth and impaired educational attainment.	Strong El Nino weather events lead to a loss of up to half of the grain harvest in South America and Africa. Both warmer water and ocean acidification affect fish stocks. A US study of long-term trends in rain, crops, food prices and migration concluded that climate change was a contributory factor to the 2010–2011 Arab Spring uprisings.
	Migration and conflict	Forced displacement has more adverse health impacts than voluntary or planned resettlement. These include malnutrition, food- and water-borne diseases, sexually transmitted diseases, diseases relating to overcrowding (measles, meningitis, acute respiratory infections), maternal mortality and mental illness.	An analysis of 234 conflicts across 175 countries in the period 1950–2004 showed the chance of civil war doubled during warm spells. El Nino events may have played a role in over 20 per cent of civil conflicts since 1950.
	Infections and vector-borne diseases	Changes in climate make environments more favourable to human pathogens, allowing more infections to occur and changes in the distribution of disease vectors.	Increases in temperature in the developing world have led to increases in campylobacter and salmonella infections. Temperature and rainfall fluctuations during 1997–1998 El Nino events resulted in expansions of: (1) breeding zones of mosquitoes carrying falciparum malaria in Kenya, (2) schistosomiasis-bearing snails in north-eastern China, (3) tick-borne encephalitis in northern Sweden and (4) Lyme disease-transmitting ixodid ticks in north-eastern Canada.
	Mental health	Psychiatric trauma due to conflict, forced migration and extreme weather includes post-traumatic stress, generalized anxiety, depression, aggression, suicide, somatoform disorders and substance misuse.	In Australia, weather-related catastrophes may affect one in five people with extreme stress, emotional injury and despair.

—————————— Activity 5.4 ——————————

This activity asks you to consider the health impacts of climate change in different settings.

Should we limit greenhouse gas emissions on a national or on a per capita basis? Is it fairer that populous countries, such as China and India, are allowed greater greenhouse gas emissions than countries with smaller populations?

What would the social, financial, ethical and environmental impacts of introducing carbon trading schemes be – where those with more money can buy 'the right to emit' from those with less money (who tend to emit less)?

Look at the health impacts of climate change given in Table 5.1. Which do you think will most severely affect LICs? Which will affect HICs? Now create a table detailing what needs to be done to either prevent these impacts from occurring (mitigation) or ensure that they cause minimal disruption (adaptation).

Comment

LICs	Mitigation	Adaptation
Water-borne diseases	Reduce emissions of greenhouse gases.	Education of the public.
	Flood defences.	Early recognition of water-borne diseases by health workers.
	Improve sanitation facilities.	Effective protocols and equipment in place in hospitals to treat water-borne diseases.
HICs	**Mitigation**	**Adaptation**
Air pollution	Reduce emissions of greenhouse gases to limit climate change.	Cleaning systems to improve indoor air quality.
	Reduce private motor vehicle use.	Educate the public (particularly those with morbidities such as heart disease and asthma) to avoid going out during peaks in poor air quality or temperature.
	Use less polluting fuels for machines and vehicles.	Ensure the early recognition and effective treatment of diseases precipitated by air pollution.

CLIMATE CHANGE AND FOOD PRODUCTION

The production and transportation of food is essential in a world where the population is set to reach nine billion people by 2050. Undernutrition has a range of impacts. Moderate effects include stunted growth and impaired brain development. In extreme cases, children die from a combination of starvation and immunosuppression. On a population level, conflict is more likely when groups of people compete for food and arable land or are forced to migrate to look for better prospects elsewhere.

Figure 5.3 shows how a fall in crop yield can lead to rises in global food prices. In HICs, consumers have to spend an increased proportion of their income on food.

In the world's LICs, more people go hungry because incomes are already insufficient to purchase an adequate range of foods to achieve good nutrition.

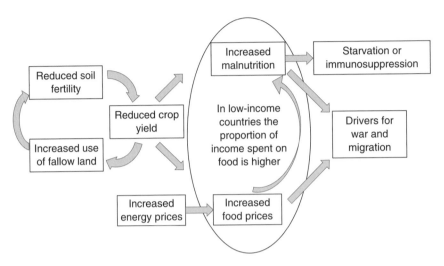

Figure 5.3   Climate change and food production

Food crop yields are sensitive to both high temperature and extreme weather. In earlier scientific models it was suggested that, while some agricultural areas would see a significant decrease in food production due to heatwaves and drought, others, especially in the global North, might benefit from warmer weather and a longer growing season. Now, however, it is expected that any benefits of a longer summer will be reversed by the effects of irregular weather – in particular, prolonged rainstorms alternating with dry weather.

Case study   Unaffordable food

In 2007, a paediatrician in a university town in Uganda, serving a large, mostly rural population, admitted a two-year-old boy with gastroenteritis, severe dehydration and severe undernutrition. His parents were subsistence farmers. The boy and his mother had travelled 18 hours, after selling livestock to pay the bus and taxi fares to reach the hospital. The boy's father had remained at home to look after the crops and the boy's four siblings. The boy was treated with IV fluids, but, because his heart was weakened by malnourishment, the fluids pushed him into acute heart failure. He died within a few hours of reaching the ward.

In the Ugandan hospital, and in many parts of sub-Saharan Africa, undernutrition is one of the most common accompanying diagnoses. Children suffering chronic undernutrition have poorly functioning immune systems, are prone to infections, and the biggest killer is acute gastroenteritis.

An audit showed that over 50 per cent of the children on this Ugandan ward met the WHO criteria for moderate undernutrition. The staff noted that admissions with undernutrition had increased between 2006 and 2007. During the same period, world cereal prices increased by

34 per cent. By 2007, parents could only afford to buy two thirds of the food they had previously been able to purchase. Food prices peaked in mid 2008 at 250 per cent of January 2006 prices.

The price spike was due to several factors, including rising oil prices (which affect the cost of mechanized production), the use of cereals to create biofuels (turning food into petrol) and market speculation. In addition, a massive drought-related crop failure was due to changing weather conditions, which are due to climate change.

CONCLUSION

In this chapter we have explored the evidence linking human health, directly and indirectly, with our environment. We have seen that science and technology can protect us from environmental hazards and have produced many of the astonishing health gains of the past century. We now also recognize that science and technology have produced large-scale environmental changes, which we struggle to manage and which will undermine many of those health gains. These new environmental hazards are inequitably distributed and it is the people who are socially, economically, culturally, politically and institutionally marginalized who are disproportionately affected by them. Fortunately, many of the actions needed to maintain ecosystem health also benefit human health. These are considered in Chapter 6.

REFERENCES

Barton, H. and Grant, M. (2006) 'A health map for the local human habitat', *Journal for the Royal Society for the Promotion of Health*, 126(6): 252–253.

IPCC (2014) *Climate Change 2014: Impacts, Adaptation, and Vulnerability. Part A: Global and Sectoral Aspects. Contribution of Working Group II to the Fifth Assessment Report of the Intergovernmental Panel on Climate Change*. New York: Cambridge University Press. Available at: https://ipcc-wg2.gov/AR5/images/uploads/WGIIAR5-PartA_FINAL.pdf (accessed 8 October 2015).

Rockström, J., Steffen, W., Noone, K. et al. (2009) 'A safe operating space for humanity', *Nature*, 461: 472–5.

Rockstrom, J., Steffen, W., Noone, K., Persson, Å., Chapin, F.S., Lambin, E.F. et al. (2009) 'A safe operating space for humanity', *Nature*, 46: 472–475.

6

CLIMATE CHANGE, LONG-TERM CONDITIONS AND SUSTAINABLE HEALTHCARE

STEFI BARNA AND SARAH WALPOLE

Chapter overview

After reading this chapter you will be able to:

- apply the concepts of primary, secondary and tertiary prevention of disease to the environmental determinants of health
- identify ways to improve population health, reduce healthcare costs and improve the environmental sustainability of health systems
- take action to improve health globally and locally.

INTRODUCTION

In Chapter 5, we discussed the fact that anthropogenic climate change is predicted to pose a major threat to human health in the twenty-first century. In this chapter, the ways in which the health sector itself contributes to global warming are considered. In the European Union, the health system produces at least 5 per cent of total CO_2 emissions, along with vast amounts of waste. If public health and the ability of future generations to meet their health needs are to be safeguarded, our use of energy and natural resources (what we buy and use) and how we manage waste in healthcare must be improved.

Reducing carbon emissions in the health sector helps to reduce the severity of climate change. New models of sustainable healthcare can also reduce the escalating rates of long-term conditions, improve the quality of care and save money.

This chapter explores how more effective prevention, management and treatment services can be delivered and advocates healthcare reforms to protect health globally and locally.

LEVELS OF PREVENTION

Imagine that you are standing by the shore of a swiftly flowing river and you hear a drowning man cry out. You jump into the cold water, fight against the strong current and force your way to the man. You grasp him tightly and swim slowly back to shore. You pull him on to the bank and start CPR. Just as he begins to revive, you hear another cry for help. You jump back into the water. You struggle against the current and eventually reach a drowning woman. You eventually get her to shore, lift her on to the bank beside the man and start to resuscitate her. Just as she begins to breathe, you hear yet another cry for help. Astonished, exhausted and overwhelmed, you return to the cold waters and force your way to a desperate child. Although the child is light, it is only with great effort that you are able to bring him to shore, lay him on the bank and start to revive him. Near exhaustion, it occurs to you that you are so busy saving people that you have no time to see what is happening 'upstream' causing them to fall into the river.

As this example suggests, identifying and acting on the root causes of injury and illness is a powerful way to prevent suffering and death. Table 6.1 gives examples of primary (upstream), secondary and tertiary levels of prevention.

Table 6.1   Levels of prevention

Levels of prevention	Types of interventions
Primary prevention (protect healthy people from disease or injury)	Education about nutrition, exercise, smoking.
	Legislation about seat belt and helmet use.
	Immunization against infectious diseases.
	Control of workplace hazards.
	Prevent contamination of water, food and air.
Secondary prevention (detect and treat disease in the early stages before it causes significant damage to health; limit long-term disability or re-injury)	Daily low-dose aspirin to prevent a second heart attack or stroke.
	Modified work tasks for injured workers.
	Antenatal screening for anaemia, high blood pressure and diabetes.
	Cervical smears and mammography to detect cancers for early intervention.
Tertiary prevention (manage long-term health problems to prevent complications and maximize quality of life)	Cardiac or stroke rehabilitation programmes.
	Chronic pain management programmes.
	Patient support groups.
	Weight control for people with diabetes, high blood pressure or arthritis.
	Regular exercise for osteoporosis.
	Prophylactic antibiotic use for chronic bronchitis and emphysema.

—————————————————————— Activity 6.1 ——————————————————————

Observe clinicians at work and notice how they introduce lifestyle changes into consultations
and treatment plans. Do they focus appropriately on primary, secondary or tertiary prevention?
What might you do differently?

Comment

Look up guidance on motivational interviewing, which can help patients make lifestyle changes
to improve their health.

Table 6.1 applies various levels of prevention to common health conditions. Is it
possible to apply different levels of protection to climate change in the same
way?

Many extreme weather events are unavoidable, due to greenhouse gases accumulated since the Industrial Revolution. Some countries have initiated measures to adapt,
such as installing flood defences to protect against storm surges, river flooding and
rises in sea level, as well as heat warning systems, to prepare for increased hospitaliza-
tions during heatwaves. These adaptation measures respond to an existing health
problem and are therefore similar to secondary prevention measures in healthcare.

A more 'upstream', or primary prevention, approach is to prevent greenhouse
gases from entering the atmosphere at all: 'mitigation of climate change'. It has
powerful protective effects and it increases health equity by offering most benefit to
the most vulnerable people (Table 6.2).

Table 6.2   Levels of prevention in climate change

Levels of prevention	Environmental interventions
Primary prevention	**Mitigation**
(protect healthy people from climate-related disease or injury)	Prevent a global temperature rise of more than 2°C by reducing greenhouse gas emissions.
Secondary prevention	**Adaptation**
(detect and treat climate-related disease in the early stages before it causes significant damage to health; limit long-term disability or re-injury)	Prepare for climate-related health threats that we cannot prevent by having emergency response teams for floods, rehousing, the social and economic disruption of community displacement, and cool rooms where heat-vulnerable patients and workers can shelter during heatwaves.
Tertiary prevention	Ensure cities are resilient and can adapt to new climate conditions and food insecurity.
(manage long-term climate-related health problems to prevent complications and maximize quality of life)	Develop food crops that thrive despite drought, flood and new pests.
	Have immigration policies in place to accommodate environmental refugees.
	Manage escalating armed conflicts over fresh water and arable land.

Activity 6.2

Most institutions have a sustainability policy. Which sustainability initiatives have been introduced in your organization?

Comment

Did you note how the policy is communicated to staff, students and service users? Are actions taken beyond simply turning off lights and computers? Who are the sustainability champions and what do they do? How are changes measured and publicized?

THE PROBLEM WITH HEALTH SERVICES

Healthcare organizations are highly resource-intensive enterprises and healthcare has itself become a major contributor to climate change. In 2008, the UK's Climate Change Act committed the government to reducing CO_2 emissions by 80 per cent by the year 2050, based on 1990 levels. This target is based on the level of emissions needed to prevent a global temperature increase of more than 2°C.

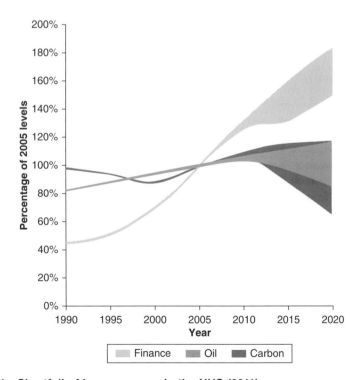

Figure 6.1   Shortfall of key resources in the NHS (2011)

Source: Reprinted with permission from NHS England Sustainable Development Unit, 2012.

In response, the National Health Service in England set about estimating the carbon footprint of the health system. It discovered that it produces one quarter of all public-sector carbon emissions, making it the largest public-sector contributor to climate change in Europe. The NHS Sustainable Development Unit was formed to ensure that the health service is, 'part of the solution, rather than part of the problem' and its Carbon Reduction Strategy set out a route map to meet the Climate Change Act's targets (NHS England Sustainable Development Unit, 2012; Roberts and Edwards, 2010)

Figure 6.1 shows the NHS's exponential growth in consumption of oil, carbon and money over the past few years and the reductions needed. In many cases, measures to reduce carbon emissions also save money. For example, installing combined heat and power in hospitals could save over £49 million and 232,000 tonnes of CO_2 per year.

Energy use in buildings, however, constitutes only a quarter of the NHS's carbon footprint. A full 16 per cent of all emissions is due to staff and patient travel. An astonishing 59 per cent comes from procurement – the purchase of goods and services, particularly pharmaceuticals. Figure 6.2 shows the carbon emissions attributable to each type of product consumed by the NHS.

Changing boilers and light bulbs alone will deliver only a small proportion of the mandated 80 per cent reduction in emissions. To achieve various targets, reductions are needed in a range of emission sources (see Figure 6.3), from estate management to clinical management and clinical care.

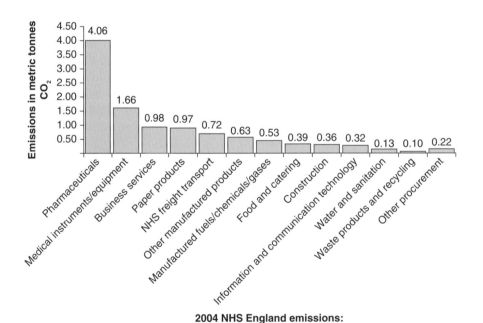

2004 NHS England emissions:
11.07 metric tonnes CO_2 procurement subsector breakdown

Figure 6.2   Emissions by procurement subcategory in the NHS

Source: NHS England Sustainable Development Unit (2012)

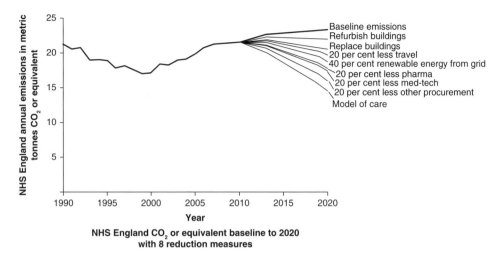

NHS England CO$_2$ or equivalent baseline to 2020
with 8 reduction measures

Figure 6.3   Potential for the NHS to effect CO$_2$ reduction

Source: NHS England Sustainable Development Unit (2010)

SUSTAINABLE HEALTHCARE

A growing body of evidence is emerging for the 'triple win' of a sustainable healthcare system: building healthier lifestyles and communities, reducing long-term conditions and increasing health equity. A sustainable healthcare system emphasizes disease prevention and health promotion, supports patients and their families to take an active role in their own care and provides 'lean' treatment services (Schroeder et al., 2012).

──────────────── Activity 6.3 ────────────────

Download *Fit for the Future* (at: www.sduhealth.org.uk/news/64/is-the-nhs-fit-for-the-future. pdf) and look at the visioning exercise for the NHS, which includes four scenarios for environmental challenges, technological advances and demographic change in 2030. Which scenario do you find the most persuasive?

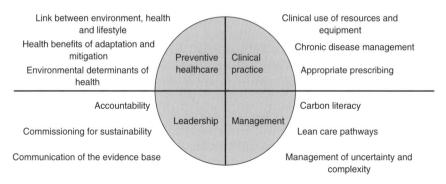

Figure 6.4   Sustainable healthcare: four action areas

Source: NHS England Sustainable Development Unit (2012)

Let's look at a few examples of what sustainability might mean for clinical practice. Figure 6.4 illustrates the key areas of preventive healthcare, clinical practice, management, leadership and advocacy.

PREVENTIVE HEALTHCARE

All healthcare activities have an environmental impact, but healthcare is only needed when people fall ill. Preventing disease reduces the need for healthcare and also reduces the suffering inherent in illness. Let's look at a few examples of prevention.

It is possible to improve population health simply by changing the way in which we produce and consume energy. Sedentary, high-carbon lifestyles are now prevalent in HICs and LMICs. The reliance on fossil fuels for transportation, food production and leisure activities reduces daily physical activity, increases high-calorie, low-nutrition diets and results in both an explosion of obesity-related conditions and a fast track to global warming.

ACTIVE TRAVEL

Physical inactivity is responsible for over three million deaths annually from cardiovascular disease, cancer and type 2 diabetes mellitus. Urban sprawl is 'obesogenic' – that is, it creates weight gain by prioritizing car use over walking and cycling.

Replacing private vehicles with 'active travel' options that make walking, cycling and public transportation the most accessible, rapid and pleasant ways to travel can reduce the burden of road traffic accidents, respiratory disease and obesity-related illness – a burden that is felt disproportionately by more disadvantaged sectors of the population (Roberts and Edwards, 2010).

ELECTRICITY AND HEALTH

Access to electricity has significantly raised living standards in industrialized countries, with a positive impact on many social determinants of health. For example, refrigeration extends the length of time that food and medications can be stored. When electricity is generated by burning fossil fuels such as coal or oil, however, the released gases and particulates have direct negative impacts on health. In China, coal-fired power plants are responsible for up to 670,000 smog-related deaths per year.

A healthier alternative is to produce electricity from sources that are renewable – that is, naturally replenished at a faster rate than we use them, such as solar, geothermal and wind power. The WHO's *Health in the Green Economy* series suggests that locally generated renewable energy can offer a more reliable source of electricity than centralized fossil fuel-burning power plants and can create jobs in a 'green economy', bringing increased employment without health hazards (WHO, 2011).

SOCIAL CAPITAL

The consumption of food, drink, private transportation and housing make up a significant proportion of our environmental impact. New collaborative forms of consumption, including car share schemes, community supported agriculture, community-based energy generation projects and local economy trading schemes all reduce the consumption and transportation of goods. They also contribute to the development of 'social capital' – the rich social and community interactions that reduce an individual's risk of dementia, depression and other illnesses.

There are many more ways in which reducing greenhouse gas emissions can benefit health. Table 6.3 lists a few of them.

Table 6.3   Health benefits of a low-carbon society

Sustainable behaviour	Direct health impacts	Impacts on social and environmental determinants of health	Policy support
Active travel	Reduces obesity, diabetes, respiratory and cardiovascular disease, some cancers, depression, osteoporosis, traffic injuries.	Decreases air pollution, including ozone, nitrous oxide and fine particulate matter. Hay fever season increases regionally due to vehicle emissions. Community cohesion and decreased street violence as a result of pedestrianized public spaces.	Education, information and motivation for patients given by health professionals: cycle training in schools and cycle awareness for motorists. Built environment: 20 mph limits, safe cycle lanes and walkways, dedicated bus lanes. Financial: fuel taxation, subsidized public transport, cycle to work schemes.
Reduce meat and dairy consumption	Diet-related cardiovascular disease, cancers, obesity.	Rearing livestock emits methane and requires more land and inputs than growing crops to provide equivalent food energy.	Dietary guidelines and nutritional labeling. Healthy eating education, such as meat-free days. Market interventions, including fiscal measures.
Insulation of buildings	Cold, damp buildings are linked to respiratory disease, mental illness and days off work.	Reduced heating costs leaves more disposable income for other expenses.	Programmes to insulate older building stock. Legislation to adequately insulate new buildings.
Reduce room temperature in buildings	Overheated rooms are linked to increased risk of infection in healthcare settings.	Excessive heating contributes to greenhouse gas levels and local air pollution from power stations.	Care Quality Commission inspection criteria for healthy temperatures.

SUSTAINABLE CLINICAL PRACTICE

Practising clinical medicine in a sustainable way requires creativity when managing long-term conditions. This includes judicious prescribing, effective use of medical technologies, non-pharmacological interventions and patient self-care. Let's consider examples from general practice and kidney care.

Case study   Greening general practice

Sally is a junior doctor who wanted to understand environmental sustainability and 'how doctors in general practice can play their part'. In a meeting at her busy, rural general practice in Somerset, she highlighted the health benefits of environmental sustainability and asked for help in identifying opportunities to improve practice. Other doctors resisted implementing sustainability plans immediately, but Sally raised the issue again in a later meeting and this time a few colleagues agreed. They started with four actions:

1. reducing the environmental impact of travel by cycling to home visits
2. conducting a waste audit to increase recycling and reduce waste
3. raising awareness with a waiting room poster
4. keeping sustainability on the practice agenda.

Sally used the sustainable action planning framework (see Activity 6.4, below) to identify performance indicators, a change strategy and an evaluation approach. She found that two thirds of her home visits over a three-month period were within one and a half miles of the practice; close enough to cycle to. She found that cycling did not take much longer than driving. In fact, closer visits were often quicker by bicycle as they avoided congestion and parking problems. She also saved the practice 45 per cent on travel costs and 0.02 CO_2e tonnes in three months (equivalent to four hours in an electric shower). There were also health benefits for Sally herself as she burned about 4160 calories over 3 months, which is equivalent to 16 chocolate bars (800g of milk chocolate).

She found cycling to home visits manageable and enjoyable. She liked the fresh air and playing her part in reducing emissions. For patients, appearing on a bicycle often raised a smile!

Individual GPs may be reluctant to cycle because of weather, low fitness levels, carrying the doctor's bag, getting sweaty en route or busy roads, but even if only a few choose to cycle occasionally – perhaps only on warm, sunny days – everyone would benefit. Practice bikes can be kept at the surgery to enable this.

To audit waste disposal, Sally collected, categorized and weighed all practice waste on one day, identified 18 categories of waste, estimated the annual amounts of waste for each category and calculated the carbon footprint of waste disposal using the Royal College of GPs' Carbon Footprinter. She found that about 65 per cent of all practice waste could be recycled and, by changing contractors, organizing recycling bins and reducing the number of collections, she saved the practice £755 (20 per cent of their spend on waste management) in the first year.

At the end of the year, Sally reflected on what she had learned about the relationship between climate change and health, sustainability and how doctors can balance responsibilities to individual patients and society:

Some practices have sustainability fully integrated into management with clear delegation of responsibilities, regular communication with the staff regarding changes and investment in green schemes. Other practices have no sustainability policy, no discussion regarding change and no consideration of energy efficiency. Many staff members are interested in environmental issues, but don't have the time or know-how to make changes. Yet, promoting carbon reduction could be one of our most important contributions to patients' health.

People's perceptions varied from intrigued to disinterested, but staff did listen and act on my suggestions. Just being there seemed to make them think and change behaviour. It is tricky to advocate for something which is poorly understood and which challenges fundamental cultural and moral issues. I realized that nothing would be achieved by dictating and demanding change. The best way is simply to make people aware of the facts. I tried not to take criticism or antagonism personally and tried to lead by example.

To learn more about the Sustainable Healthcare GP Registrar Scholarship, read Sally Aston's 'How to' guide (at: http://sustainablehealthcare.org.uk/sustainable-primary-care/resources/2012/03/making-change-towards-sustainability-sustainable-action-p).

──────────── Activity 6.4   Sustainable action planning ────────────

Sustainable action planning (SAP) is a framework to support clinical teams that want to focus their priorities and put together a green action plan. Watch the short video about the Green Nephrology project in kidney care (at: http://sustainablehealthcare.org.uk/sustainable-specialties-greening-nephrology). This is an excellent example of how to improve clinical outcomes and the patient experience, while minimizing low-value activity, such as travel, and addressing the 'triple bottom line' of quality, cost and environmental sustainability. Using the Green Nephrology example, design a SAP for your setting (see: http://sap.sustainablehealthcare.org.uk).

Comment

Your SAP might include some of the following suggestions.

- Avoid overdiagnosis – that is, think twice before ordering investigations that may be unnecessary, waste resources and potentially expose patients to harm.
- Prescribe appropriately – nearly 30 per cent of the NHS' carbon footprint comes from prescription medicines. A 10 per cent reduction in pharmaceutical wastage would lower overall health service emissions by 2 per cent and save significant sums that could be used for other interventions. Where pharmaceuticals are indicated, using oral drugs over intravenous ones saves financial and natural resources.
- Work interprofessionally – ask your pharmacy for its sustainable procurement plans, for example.
- Prescribe exercise when indicated – the benefits of physical activity to health, longevity and protection from illness can surpass the effectiveness of drugs in some cases.
- Consider care in the community – care close to home and planned, timely discharges save money and carbon.
- Plan use of medical equipment. Before performing procedures, consider which disposable items you are going to use – only open packets that you know will be needed, opening others only as necessary. This saves resources and carbon and can reduce the risk of transmitting infections.

(Continued)

(Continued)

- Avoid printing – the carbon cost of producing, transporting and recycling or shredding paper is significant. Reducing the printing of patient information also protects confidentiality.
- Procure ethically – ask your supplies department to source recycled products where available.
- Talk to patients – use interactions with patients to promote healthy, sustainable choices.

MANAGEMENT, LEADERSHIP AND ADVOCACY

Public trust in traditional leaders (politicians, corporations and media) is in grave decline, but health practitioners have largely managed to retain public trust and patients continue to value their opinions on matters that pertain to human health. Given their trusted position in society and responsibility to protect and improve health nationally and internationally, healthcare professionals and students can take a powerful leadership role in bringing about a more equitable and healthier world. Wherever you are in your healthcare career, the decisions you make will help to shape the face of the healthcare system and society that you will be working in for decades to come. Health professionals have an important function, as advocates for health, as leaders and as role models for colleagues, patients and the public. In a clinical environment, they can improve practice so that limited resources are used responsibly.

Healthcare professionals are responsible to patients, the public and communities and to the children and future grandchildren of those communities. Here are some of the ways in which health professionals can contribute to the management of a sustainable healthcare system.

- Knowledge
  - Explore how NHS leaders manage uncertainty and complexity in a changing health service and learn from the most thoughtful and creative people.
  - Become carbon literate and learn to communicate the evidence base on climate change and health, both formally and informally (see Activity 6.5, below, to practise your skills).

- Personal actions
  - Model appropriate behaviour by, for instance, setting up or joining a car pool, using active transport, avoiding flying when possible, reducing meat and dairy consumption, switching off equipment when not in use.
  - Tackle waste – set up recycling in shared areas, implement measures to avoid sterile equipment being opened unless it is definitely going to be used, and investigate whether or not autoclaving (heat cleaning) of instruments is used in your hospital.
  - Make meetings and travel more sustainable – reduce travel by using telephone and video conferencing, encourage the drinking of tap water rather than bottled and provide sustainably sourced, vegetarian food.

- Sustainability planning in healthcare
  - Ask your dean or estates department for their sustainability plans.
  - Ask your trust or surgery to show how it practises sustainable commissioning.
  - Challenge conference organizers to adopt more sustainable meetings.

o One in 20 journeys on UK roads is related to the NHS! Ask your medical school or training organization to devise a sustainable placement policy to minimize travel while maximizing training opportunities.

o Promote active travel or write exercise prescriptions for conditions that would otherwise require carbon-intensive pharmaceutical treatment.

o Ask placement and rota coordinators to set timetables that allow you to use public transport wherever possible and study/work from home, if feasible (this could also improve your work–life balance).

- Awareness and advocacy beyond healthcare

  o Speak to the media about policies that have benefits to health as well as ecological sustainability. Inform employers or clinical staff as needed. Lobby your local council, MPs and professional or student organization to promote health and sustainability (see Activity 6.5).

Activity 6.5

A sustainable healthcare practitioner understands the links between environment, health and lifestyle and the health benefits of climate change adaptation and mitigation policies. Advocating these approaches requires good communication skills. Test your understanding of this chapter by using a variety of communication styles to explain the key issues.

1. Take an informal, conversational approach. Speak to someone about what you have understood from this chapter and Chapter 5. Use the list of points below or make your own, but try to keep your 'story' to five minutes or less. Afterwards, note down which parts of your explanation seemed to go over well or badly and why you think that might be. Then ask the person for his or her impressions of the conversation and what you might have done more effectively. Use the feedback to triangulate your assessment of your skills. If possible, have another go with a new interlocutor. This is called informal advocacy and it forms an important part of doctors' health advocacy.

2. Try out a formal proposal. Set up a similar discussion with a friendly faculty member or supervising clinician. Take just a few of your points, make them more concise and ask for an action or outcome. Your conversation should take no more than two to three minutes. Reflect again on what worked and ask for feedback. You may be asked to put your thoughts into writing for further consideration.

3. Put it in writing. Write a brief letter to an influential person in the media, government or health management. Focus on clear, concise messages and state what actions you as a healthcare professional would recommend.

Comment

Key messages are listed below. Keep practising and refining your communication skills and you will be surprised to see how positively people begin to respond.

- The health of the environment is linked to human health and can support or undermine our ability to protect and promote the health of patients and the public.
- Healthcare provision has environmental impacts that affect health locally (such as air pollution) and globally (such as climate change).

(Continued)

(Continued)

- Lifestyle behaviours – including travel, diet and consumption habits – that are good for an individual's health often also have positive environmental impacts.
- Health inequity can be exacerbated or ameliorated by environmental and climate change policies.
- Good management in healthcare requires carbon literacy.
- 'Lean' care pathways use resources as efficiently as possible and provide high quality patient care.
- Good managers respond appropriately to uncertainty and complexity, including the unpredictable health consequences of climate change.

CONCLUSION

Clinical care contributes to environmental degradation through the use of resources (mainly water, raw materials and fossil fuels) and production of waste (especially greenhouse gases from waste incineration and landfill). Powerful synergies exist, however, between practices that promote environmental sustainability and those that promote health. Reducing greenhouse gas emissions and moving towards a low-carbon society will bring substantial health benefits everywhere, including in industrialized countries. The greatest health benefits will accrue from early, rather than delayed, carbon reduction measures.

The NHS's plan to reduce carbon emissions by 80 per cent by 2050 will have a major impact on the health service that you will work in. Recent healthcare graduates are likely to lead the move to a sustainable healthcare service. Health professionals have an important role to play in reducing environmental degradation from health service activities, through effective use of technologies, appropriate information management, minimizing low-value activities and use of natural resources (non-pharmacological) and human resources (self-care). Look for approaches that are a 'win-win' for both health and the environment.

FURTHER INFORMATION

- The Sustainable Development Unit works with UK healthcare professionals to develop guidance regarding ways to improve sustainability in healthcare settings. www.sduhealth.org.uk
- The Centre for Sustainable Healthcare develops programmes to measure and reduce the environmental footprint of medical and surgical specialties. www.sustainablehealthcare.org.uk
- The Climate and Health Council has resources for health professionals. www.climateandhealth.org
- For a humorous approach to understanding 'carbon dependence syndrome'. www.carbonaddict.org

REFERENCES

National Health Service (2011) *Update: NHS Carbon Reduction Strategy for England.* Available at: www.sdu.nhs.uk/documents/publications/UPDATE_NHS_Carbon_Reduction_ Strategy_(web).pdf (accessed 8 October 2015).

National Health Service for England Sustainable Development Unit (2010) *CO2e Reduction Potential* for *NHS England: GHG Emissions 2010–2020 Reduction Measures Update.* Available at: www.sduhealth.org.uk/resources/default.aspx?q=cO2 (accessed 27 October 2015).

National Health Service for England Sustainable Development Unit (2012) *Sustainability in the NHS: Health Check.* Cambridge: NHS Sustainable Development Unit. Available at: www.sduhealth.org.uk/resources/default.aspx?q=sustainability+in+the+nhs+2012 (accessed 8 October 2015).

Roberts, I. and Edwards, P. (2010) *The Energy Glut: The Politics of Fatness in an Overheating World.* London: Zed Books.

Schroeder, K., Thompson, T., Frith, K. and Pencheon, D. (2012) *Sustainable Healthcare.* BMJ Books. Chichester: John Wiley and Sons.

World Health Organization (2011) *Health in the Green Economy.* Available at: www.who. int/hia/hgebrief_health.pdf (accessed 8 October 2015).

PART III
GLOBAL HEALTH IN PRACTICE

7

WORKING WITH MIGRANTS, REFUGEES AND ASYLUM SEEKERS

PHILIP COTTON AND ANDREA WILLIAMSON

Chapter overview

After reading this chapter you will be able to:

- explain the causes of migration
- describe how cultural and social factors can affect physical and mental health
- explain issues affecting access to health services
- describe the roles of social care, the voluntary sector and the community in relation to migrants
- apply practical solutions.

INTRODUCTION

The migration of people across continents, countries and communities is determined by history, economics and conflict. Over time, patterns of migration change, as do sociopolitical attitudes and controls. Successive waves to and from the UK have produced the diverse communities and rich cultural landscape that constitutes the country today.

This chapter is about migrant health in the early twenty-first century and sets out a brief overview of migration, then focuses on the health and healthcare of migrants who have sought asylum, those who have been accepted as refugees and those who have been refused asylum (RAS) in the UK. Because of the diversity and complexity of socio-geopolitical and healthcare contexts involved, this chapter cannot provide an overview of all migrant groups in the UK or elsewhere.

--------- Activity 7.1 ---------

Go to Oxford University's Migration Observatory (at: www.migrationobservatory.ox.ac.uk/briefings/
immigration-detention-uk) and make notes on what information you can locate from this portal
about immigration detention facilities in the UK.

Comment

The UK is able to detain 3500 people in its facilities at any one time. Nearly half of detainees are
seeking asylum. They are detained to establish identity, assess their claim, facilitate deportation
or because there are concerns about risks of absconding. Since 2005, detention has also been
used to help fast-track some applicants. Around 29,000 people were detained in 2012, most
for under two months.

OVERVIEW OF MIGRATION

Migration is viewed increasingly as a major global health challenge. About one billion people are either internal or international migrants worldwide (WHO, 2013).
Migration is not the simple movement of people from their place of origin to new
ones. Migration is now viewed as a process that has five stages, described as,
'pre-departure, travel, destination, interception, and return'. These stages influence
migrants' health, both positively and negatively. Their health is affected by the setting at their point of origin, their experiences en route and the determinants of
health in the setting in which they settle. The traditional approach to migration
within silos, such as security, trade or aid, is not fit for purpose and a global,
integrated approach is required (Zimmerman and Kiss, 2011).

This chapter takes account of individual patients within their families and
communities, using knowledge from medicine, social sciences and geopolitics,
and galvanizing professional and community groups to utilize skill sets as diverse
as clinical problemsolving, legal advice and community development. A rights-
based ethical perspective is taken, drawing on the literature and experience of
working as primary care clinicians with asylum seekers, refugees and 'refused
asylum seekers' (RAS).

ASYLUM SEEKERS, REFUGEES AND RAS

Asylum seekers apply for protection as refugees. Refugees flee their countries due
to well-founded fear of persecution there. The UK adheres to UN and European
agreements on refugees and human rights and so cannot return asylum applicants
to a place where they are likely to face torture or persecution. In 2011, persons
applying for asylum were an estimated 7 per cent of net migration to the UK (0.41
asylum applicants per 1000 of the population). Of applicants in the UK, 33 per
cent were granted 'leave to remain'. Of the negative decisions appealed, 22 per cent
of those subsequently were accepted. Since 1994, the majority of decisions have
been refusals.

CULTURAL CONTEXT

Migrants bring their own health beliefs that are influenced by gender roles, social setting, faith background, education, employment background and national and or tribal cultural health practices. To varying degrees over time (the evidence is conflicting), migrants adopt the health beliefs and behaviours of the communities and cultures they encounter in the UK. Thus, trying to predict and understand why patients present with symptoms, what those symptoms might mean, how patients may respond to information and interact with the healthcare system in the UK is complex.

It is important for healthcare workers to have an overview of factors having a significant impact on the health of some migrant patients. These include female genital cutting and regional patterns of violence (Freedom from Torture, 2014; Human Rights Watch, 2014). Historically, the mental health field is the most sensitive to culturally bound ideas about what constitutes mental illness (see Chapter 11). In our experience, however, although learning about broad principles and topic areas are important, key learning comes from talking with patients and utilizing the expertise of interpreters who come from a cultural background similar to that of the patient with whom you are both working.

SOCIAL CONTEXT

Currently, when people make asylum applications, they are allocated accommodation in a city and area chosen by the UK Border Agency representatives, receive minimum benefits and are not allowed to take up employment. So, individuals have to adjust to a new culture and make new social contacts within the constraints of a very limited income, with no opportunity to take up paid employment.

Activity 7.2

Reflect on what these constraints mean for the people experiencing them. List your thoughts.

Comment

In our experience, this is difficult for most people who are used to earning and deriving social benefits from working or having a role within a community. Individuals have to live with the uncertainty of their citizenship status as they go through the asylum process. Moreover, the process itself is experienced as negative when describing personal, often traumatic and sometimes shameful experiences in an environment seeking to disprove the case the person is putting forward (Mulvey, 2013). There is limited evidence that the asylum process has a greater negative impact on people's mental well-being than the previous traumatic experiences in their countries of origin (Papadopoulos et al., 2010).

All of these social and system factors lead to asylum seekers experiencing high levels of stress and although, in our experience, most asylum seekers demonstrate high levels of personal resilience, when these are combined with the problems of day-to-day life, worries about family members and ongoing conflicts in their countries of origin, these people then become ill.

Once people have a positive decision and are granted 'leave to remain', a further dislocation can occur. Although, with refugee status, comes the ability to work, refugees often have difficulty obtaining higher-paid jobs and experience in-work poverty (Lindsay, Gillespie and Dobbie, 2010). Housing provision often changes, too, and refugees have to start to navigate the complex social housing system. They may have to move to a different area, which weakens any social networks they have built up. Moreover, only a minority of refugees have permanent leave to remain (and, hence, can become citizens) in the UK – the majority continue to live with the uncertainty of their leave being revoked, which is another barrier to securing long-term employment (Gillespie, 2012).

If a person's asylum application is refused, an unknown number of people either opt to or are required to stay on in the UK because it is not safe to return to their country of origin. Refused asylum seeker (RAS) status means 'no recourse to public funds'. Access to state benefits, housing and (in all countries in the UK except Scotland) to healthcare, apart from immediate and necessary treatment, is denied. The Scottish government, however, ruled in 2012 that all people who had ever lodged an asylum application were eligible to access all NHS services, no matter what their current citizenship status. RAS in the UK fall below the global UN poverty target income of $1.25 per day (Gillespie, 2012). Numbers of people who are RAS are unknown because the UK Border Agency does not collect data about them.

MENTAL HEALTH

There is most evidence to draw on in the health research literature about the mental health of asylum seekers, refugees and RAS.

Activity 7.3

List some possible reasons for this being the case.

Comment

The best available information about this to date is from a systematic review of the prevalence of mental illness in refugees in Western countries (Fazel, Wheeler and Danesh, 2005). The authors noted heterogeneity across all the studies they included due to differences in study designs, tools used and populations studied. They concluded that the most important finding is the prevalence of post-traumatic stress disorder is about ten times more common in refugees than it is in the general population. A possible reason for this finding could be the new challenges that asylum seekers, refugees and RAS brought to the health services in the global North, their accounts of detention, torture, witnessing the death of family members, sexual exploitation and systematic rape manifesting as psychological symptoms.

Post-traumatic stress disorder is the term used to describe the psychological symptoms experienced by individuals who have been exposed to traumatic events that provoked intense fear, helplessness and horror. Individuals go on to relive these traumas through flashbacks, intrusive thoughts or nightmares. Triggers prompting them to relive the traumas are avoided, leading to a state of increased psychological arousal. Exposure to a one-off traumatic event, such as a terrorist attack or sexual attack, is a Type 1 trauma. Type 2 or complex trauma is when individuals are exposed to a series of traumatic events, such as those already described, or have experienced significant adverse events at developmentally important times in their lives. This can bring about additional significant impairment in terms of dissociation, emotional dysregulation, somatic distress and relational alienation. Treatment options include the use of medication and psychological therapy work, often focused on a range of trauma therapy. Helping individuals to feel safe in their body, emotions, relationships and environment is important and helps explain why the asylum application process can have such a negative impact on health.

PHYSICAL HEALTH

Historically, the physical health needs of migrants have been approached from a public health perspective considering the illnesses that migrants may import to their destination country (Gushulak and MacPherson, 2006). Health screening for migrants at port of entry still operates from this perspective. As health services for asylum seekers, refugees and RAS are focused on a rights-based approach to effective healthcare, however, the question is more accurately, which prevalent health conditions must health professionals need to be competent in identifying and treating in order to best promote the health of their patients? Answering this question is not straightforward due to the great heterogeneity between migrant populations and their contexts.

--- Activity 7.4 ---

Find out what the physical health needs are for your local area by looking at the most recent health needs assessment you can find.

Comment

Though we cannot guess what you were able to discover about your area, we can provide a framework from which to consider which physical health issues are important for an asylum seeker, refugee or RAS in the UK.

Framework for understanding and managing health needs

- What is the presenting problem(s)?
- Stop: do we need an interpreter for this to be an effective consultation?
- Which knowledge and skills are needed for every patient presenting with this problem?
- Which additional knowledge and skills might I need to employ, taking into account this specific patient's sociocultural context?
- Which interventions might help? (Medical, self-help, advocacy.)

It is useful to consider what physical health needs are important to patients who are seeking asylum, are refugees or who are RAS in addition to those experienced by the general population. They may present with the same health problems (respiratory, musculoskeletal, cardiovascular, dermatological) as any other patient, but, because of the specific regional, country, tribal, social or political context these patients may have experienced at the start of their migration from a country or context they may have travelled through, specific health diagnoses or solutions may be required. Consider, for example, schistosomiasis in the differential diagnosis of haematuria with a patient from sub-Saharan Africa; complex trauma in the form of abdominal pain in a patient who was detained and tortured in Iraq; or health beliefs about taking long-term medication in the ongoing treatment of high blood pressure with a patient who comes from a rural Afghanistani setting with no written literacy skills. This situation is illustrated by the following case study.

Case study

AB is a 23-year-old woman from the Horn of Africa who is currently living in a hostel for homeless people. She has refugee status. She presents to her GP with difficulty sleeping and heartburn.

Which history and examination areas would you wish to cover?

First of all, establish whether or not an interpreter is required. This patient feels confident in spoken and medical English.

Which questions would you ask every patient who gave the above history?

- **Sleep** Time frame, what is normal, triggers (include pain), depression screen, sleep hygiene. It is over three weeks since the patient moved to the hostel. She is worried about the future, feels lonely, but otherwise is well. Previously, she slept eight hours per night, but now she has about five hours' broken sleep.
- **Heartburn** Time frame, triggers, red flags, past history, smoking, alcohol. She has experience heartburn for the past three weeks, there has been a change in diet, but no red flags, she is a non-smoker and does not drink alcohol.

Which additional questions would you consider asking this patient?

- Sensitively enquire about the patient's reason for leaving the Horn of Africa and her experience of the journey to the UK, including whether or not she was detained or experienced/witnessed violence that had a negative impact. She left because she did not wish to participate in military service. Nothing of concern happened en route.
- Enquire about AB's current social circumstances, plans for the future. AB had to leave UKBA accommodation and a network of friends to move to her current hostel. She finds it noisy and feels personally threatened and is a target of racial abuse by some other residents. AB has no cooking facilities in her room and so has to buy local take-away food. This makes her feel ill and she runs short of money quickly so she struggles to keep in contact with her friends.

Conduct an abdominal examination, paying attention to signs of abdominal tenderness. Everything seems normal.

What intervention(s) would you offer?

- Acknowledge the current difficulty of AB's circumstances and the effect this is having on her. Offer appropriate sleep hygiene advice and short-term medication to alleviate dyspepsia. Talk over advocacy options – having a key worker in the hostel, input from a housing officer, having third-sector advocacy support (such as Shelter or Refugee Council). Discuss other activities that might help rebuild her social networks, to help address her safety concerns, and suggest a move to more appropriate short- and long-term accommodation.

ACCESS TO HEALTH SERVICES

ORIENTATION TO THE UK SETTING

Being new to a town or city can mean people are socially isolated. Also, they may have difficulty knowing how and where to access the most appropriate health and social services, so they may avoid seeking help or try to follow the rules that applied in their previous experiences of services. When things go wrong, they might not realize why.

If asylum seekers make contact with a local GP (family medicine) practice, language can become a barrier to registering with a doctor or understanding what entitlements there are. In some UK cities, this has been recognized. For example, in Glasgow, all arrivals who are seeking asylum are allocated to a GP practice and have an initial assessment and signposting undertaken by an Asylum Bridging Team. While asylum seekers may come from resource-poor countries, it is important to remember that people also arrive from countries where there may be direct access to high-technology tests that are not so immediately available in the NHS. Many people flee with nothing and rarely, if ever, will people arrive with their health records.

BARRIERS ENCOUNTERED IN THE UK'S HEALTH SERVICES

Structural problems in the NHS exacerbate difficulties that asylum seekers may have accessing healthcare. Poor coordination of those services frequently needed by asylum seekers is compounded by a lack of awareness of issues such as complex healthcare needs, culture, language and knowledge of various entitlements, at all levels, from frontline reception and administrative staff to health service managers and professionals. Lack of funding and facilities for services such as interpreting and public attitudes to asylum seekers are further constraints.

Cultural differences in the relationships between patients and doctors exist around the world. Doctors can be viewed as people of status, whose opinions and actions aren't questioned. Principles such as confidentiality can have different meanings in different political and social contexts and decisionmaking, which tends to focus on the individual patient in the UK, in some other cultures may be a shared family process. For some people, it may be difficult to trust doctors and other professionals because of previous associations with imprisonment and torture, when doctors were perceived to have colluded with state police or prison authorities.

HEALTHCARE DELIVERY MODELS

Feldman (2006) proposes a framework for planning services driven by the needs of asylum seekers and identifies several key components that need to be addressed when planning, monitoring and evaluating services.

Activity 7.5

Think for a moment about what you would need from a health service in a foreign country – if you were skiing in a popular resort, for example.

Comment

You might reasonably expect that the local healthcare facility could manage fractures and had arrangements to evacuate casualties to larger facilities. Why should our health service in the UK be any less responsive to asylum seekers' healthcare needs?

Asylum seekers need access to health assessments and screening and may ultimately need access to specialist hospital care. Feldman (2006) outlines three objectives for a systems approach to comprehensive healthcare for asylum seekers: enabling access, comprehensive provision and essential support services.

Access to services can be facilitated by someone working in the community who provides information about health services and can then direct people to register in primary care (in the UK, general practice). Care can be offered through mainstream general practices with tailored or enhanced services and dedicated, specially designed general practices. Whichever system of general practice is locally available, people need to be offered access to routine services, such as immunizations and screening programmes, which should be available soon after they have been housed.

Comprehensive provision of care requires the coordination and planning of services with social services and housing. This should be needs- and data-driven and will ultimately involve training for those working across these sectors and agencies. Many local organizations and several national charities provide refuge, advocacy, train healthcare workers and offer focused services supporting people who need to trace families, people with mental health problems and people who have been tortured. In the future, patient-held records may facilitate the coordination of care between different agencies in what may be quite complex cases. These patient-held records may build trust as patients know what is being written about them, though they may need to have this explained to them if they cannot read English.

WORKING WITH INTERPRETERS

IMPORTANCE

We have identified that language and communication are key components of the effective delivery of healthcare and other services. The provision of interpreting services is the main component of this.

PRACTICAL ISSUES

The NHS operates an interpreting service that includes access to a telephone service, which can be used without prior booking, and face-to-face interpreting, which needs to be scheduled. This service provides culturally sensitive interpreters who are independent of the patients/clients, their families and the healthcare or social services professionals.

A fully resourced interpreting service is crucial, as using family members and others known to the patient can constrain the consultation. Indeed, one of the warning signs that raises the question of trafficking of vulnerable individuals is close supervision by a 'family member' who accompanies the patient as interpreter.

There are three stages in effective working with interpreters: a briefing before the consultation proper, the meeting or consultation itself and a debriefing. The briefing is about introducing people to one other and being clear about the roles of the three people in the consultation.

During the consultation, the interpreter is usually tasked with interpreting word for word and, thus, in the first person. If clarification is needed, by either the interpreter or the professional, then this is conducted word for word in both languages. The client and professional sit facing in direct communication with one another, while the interpreter sits slightly out of sight, usually in a triangle pattern, in order that neither the client nor professional address the interpreter directly.

After the consultation or meeting, there is usually a debriefing to make sure that none of the parties has unresolved concerns about the process or content. This also provides an opportunity to provide a level of support for the interpreter, who may have witnessed an emotionally difficult consultation.

SOCIAL CARE

Social workers provide social support and services for patients seeking asylum and refugees in the same way that they would for UK citizens. They have a key role in supporting unaccompanied minors – that is, children who have arrived in the UK without families to care for them. There is reported tension, however, between the human rights, social justice-based approach on which social work ethics and practice are based and the statutory reporting role that social workers have with the UK Home Office (Fell and Fell, 2013; Humphries, 2004).

THE VOLUNTARY SECTOR

The voluntary sector fulfils two distinct roles in the support of migrants. The first is a campaigning role, gathering evidence, lobbying government and other decision-making bodies about the many issues that migrants face in the UK. The second is to augment or fill in any gaps in the statutory services (Wren, 2007). This is of particular importance to people who have had their asylum applications refused (Jones and Williamson, 2014) as they then become ineligible for support from the local authorities and other statutory services.

What is the evidence?

The role of the voluntary sector and the community

Glasgow night shelter

A group of voluntary organizations in Glasgow provide a night shelter for people who have had their asylum applications refused and are destitute. The shelter is open every night from 10 p.m. until 9 a.m. to provide warm, safe sleeping accommodation, food and advice about other services for people who have nowhere else to go. Most of the staff are volunteers and the setting is a church hall.

Bridging the Gap

Bridging the Gap runs a drop-in lunchtime session once a week, which includes activities and lunch. A team of volunteers from a range of backgrounds (including some who are currently seeking asylum) provide the hospitality, including cooking a lunch reflecting their cultural backgrounds. They cater for around 60 people each week. It is a tasty, noisy, friendly experience. Many people find it a positive addition to their week's activities, make friends and learn about their neighbours, who were born all over the world, including the Gorbals, in Glasgow.

COMMUNITY

People seeking asylum are housed in social housing contracted by the UK government to local authorities. This has meant that people have often been housed in more deprived city communities. When people are granted leave to remain, many continue in social housing due to having low incomes (Mulvey, 2013).

Reports of violence against people seeking asylum have been reported in the press, but so too have individuals and communities coming together to combat threats such as dawn raids to remove asylum-seeking families to detention centres. Migrants describe the feeling of belonging to a community as an important aspect of integration and this can be through neighbours and friendships as well as community-based organizations (Mulvey, 2013). Bridging the Gap is a Glasgow-based organization that was originally set up to combat Catholic/Protestant sectarian tensions, but has now widened its remit to include wider community integration for all.

TRAFFICKING AND SLAVERY

The number of women, men and children who are trafficked across borders and continents is increasing. Trafficking is distinct from smuggling. In the latter, the relationship with the smuggler ends on arrival at the destination. In trafficking, the relationship with the trafficker (commonly termed the facilitator) continues as the purpose is often for exploitation in the destination country.

Trafficking is the third most profitable illegal industry after drugs and arms (UNODC, 2012) and some of the features that make it so are a direct result of the exploitation of others. The UN is coordinating data and, in 2003, documented 460 trafficking flows involving over 100 countries, domestic, transcontinental and regional (cross-border). A 'flow' is defined as at least five people being routed this way. Around one third of all persons identified are victims of domestic trafficking (occurring within one country).

WHO IS TRAFFICKED?

Women and girls account for 75 per cent of all trafficked people, while 27 per cent are children, two-thirds of them being girls. The majority of cases of trafficking were for:

- sexual exploitation (58 per cent)
- forced labour (36 per cent)
- begging, forced marriage, illegal adoption, military conscription, debt bondage and crime (6 per cent).

A smaller but significant number of people are trafficked for removal of organs (documented in 16 countries). The most vulnerable of those trafficked are young children, women, who are often less empowered, would-be migrants looking for opportunities, newly arrived migrants, adolescents, disabled people and those isolated through poverty, discrimination and absence of roots, connections and associations. The political situation, wars and the absence of legal protection for children and minority groups also create vulnerability.

Patterns emerge in the groups of people from particular countries that are trafficked for a certain purpose and these change as soon as authorities begin to gather intelligence and clamp down on that trafficking activity. While the perpetrators of trafficking are typically male compatriots, trafficking is a crime that has a relatively high proportion of women who are given particular roles. Women involved in trafficking are more likely to get caught than their male counterparts.

ACTION

In the UK a multi-agency response is needed as trafficked children are often abused mentally, physically and sexually, so action needs to be taken involving local authority children's services, the police, NSPCC, social workers, health and sexual healthcare, mental health services, family tracing services and legal support.

PRACTICAL TIPS FOR HEALTH PROFESSIONALS

There must be early identification and recognition of children considered to be trafficked or at risk of being trafficked. Trafficked children can enter the UK legally, UK-born children may be trafficked within the UK and children can sometimes be trafficked through several countries before arriving here. It is known that children originally trafficked as domestic labour may go on to become exploited for sex. Some trafficked children will be coerced into presenting themselves as unaccompanied asylum-seeking children (UASC) and do so under continuing threat. It is known that these children will appear to settle into local authority care and schooling, but will subsequently disappear without warning. All these situations require close working relationships between the judicial service, police, immigration, health, education and social services in the UK.

All healthcare, education, and social/community workers also need to be aware of the profiles and possibilities that exist within the area of child trafficking and risk factors that can alert them to the possibility of trafficking in any one case. There needs to be a series of local authority mechanisms in place that can be brought into play as required. Several local authorities and health boards have a list of indicators (a risk assessment matrix) that helps to identify whether or not a child has been trafficked or is at risk of trafficking.

SELF-CARE FOR PROFESSIONALS AND VOLUNTEERS

Working with people who have traumatic histories is 'emotion work' and can have a significant impact on professionals, service providers or volunteers and this can lead to health problems, variously termed as burnout, secondary trauma, secondary traumatic stress, indirect trauma, compassion stress, compassion fatigue and vicarious traumatization. This often happens over a period of time and the result is behavioural change in an individual. It also has an effect on organizations. There is an unfortunate stigma attached to burnout that can be wrongly associated with individual weakness, but the greatest predictor of secondary trauma is exposure to the work.

One additional way to reduce the burden of caring is to increase one's knowledge of the area and associated problems. This can lead to an increased ability to help clients appropriately, decreases (unintentional) damage done to clients by practitioners and increases one's ability to self-care. Other ways include introducing boundaries for roles, time for rest and relaxation, reassessing priorities of work and ensuring that people have social and family lives.

Working with any specific group of people who face victimization, trauma and terror can also be hugely rewarding and the term 'compassion satisfaction' has been coined for this. Such work brings greater meaning and sense to the lives of those who care and serve.

Reducing the burden of caring and the risk of secondary trauma is something that both organizations and individuals need to respond to. To leave this with individuals is to suggest that the ability to cope is down to the individual and inappropriately places failure to cope with them. Instead, organizations need to be aware of the possibility and provide supportive facilities and access to training. Supervision, shared consulting and debriefings should be a part of the organization's culture.

For individuals, a greater self-awareness of personal behaviours that come to the fore when they are stressed is important. Achieving balance in life's activities is key and being aware of situations in which the time spent on negative and positive emotions is out of balance is helpful.

HEALTH TOURISM

A UK government consultation at the end of 2013 concluded that there should be a system of charging temporary migrants for healthcare and better systems for recognizing temporary migrants at the point of treatment and fee recovery.

The suggestion that healthcare professionals identify people who are not entitled to care, control access to it and, in so doing, restrict access to treatment is morally unacceptable to many professionals who do not wish to police this.

It is appropriate to include 'health tourism' in this chapter on asylum seekers, however, as it is an area riddled with misunderstandings and wrongly conflated with reasons for people seeking asylum in the UK.

Health tourism is when a person travels to another country with the sole intention of getting healthcare. It is an international business far bigger than the reported use of the NHS by people not entitled to do so. Agents advertise and facilitate health tourism and as many as 50 countries have a health tourism industry for procedures such as cosmetic and hip replacement surgery. The UK is a net exporter of people who obtain procedures performed overseas. That is, the number exceeds the number of people who come to the UK to have procedures performed. Also, the number of private overseas patients who come to the UK exceeds the number of UK residents who are treated privately here. Travelling overseas for private procedures raises issues of quality of care, insurance and liability, as well as pre- and post-operative care – who does it and where is it done? That includes the management of complications.

CONCLUSIONS

Shifting patterns of migration around the world mean that many countries are now comprised of multicultural communities, within which all health professionals need to be able to work. Migration is one of the world's health challenges, not simply because economic migration can leave countries under-resourced in terms of health workers but also huge pressures can be put to bear on governments, health systems and individual professionals due to war, famine and climate change when waves of migrants seek a home.

Working with people who are seeking asylum, are refugees or have had their asylum application refused, involves utilising a range of knowledge and skills, including that professionals recognise and manage the potential emotional toll of this work. It encourages clinicians to problem solve at the level of the community, family and the individual and encapsulates the multidisciplinary strength of global health work in all corners of the UK and beyond.

USEFUL SOURCES

Human Rights Watch (2014) www.hrw.org/publications

Freedom from Torture Publications (2014) www.freedomfromtorture.org/what-we-do/17/publications

REFERENCES

Fazel, M., Wheeler, J. and Danesh, J. (2005) 'Prevalence of serious mental disorder in 7000 refugees resettled in Western countries: a sytematic review', *The Lancet*, 365: 1309–14.

Feldman, R. (2006) 'Primary healthcare for refugees and asylum seekers: a review of the literature and a framework for services', *Public Health*, 120: 809–816.

Fell, B. and Fell, P. (2013) 'Welfare across borders: a social work process with adult asylum seekers', *The British Journal of Social Work*, 2013.

Freedom from Torture Publications (2014) www.freedomfromtorture.org/what-we-do/17/publications (accessed 8 October 2015).

Gillespie, M. (2012) *Trapped: Destitution and Asylum in Scotland*. UK: Refugee Survival Trust, British Red Cross and Scottish Refugee Council.

Gushulak, B.D. and MacPherson, D.W. (2006) 'The basic principles of migration health: population mobility and gaps in disease prevalence', *Emerging Themes in Epidemiology*, 3: 3.doi:10.1186/1742-7622-3-3.

Human Rights Watch (2014) www.hrw.org/publications (accessed 8 October 2015).

Humphries, B. (2004) 'An unacceptable role for social work: implementing immigration policy', *British Journal of Social Work*, 34: 93–107.

Jones, C. and Williamson, A.E. (2014) 'Volunteers working to support migrants in Glasgow: a qualitative study', *International Journal of Migration, Health and Social Care* 10(4): 193–206. doi:10.1108/IJMHSC-10-2013-0034

Lindsay, K., Gillespie, M. and Dobbie, L. (2010) *Refugees Experiences and Views of Poverty in Scotland*. UK: Scottish Refugee Council and Scottish Poverty Information Unit, Glasgow Caledonian University.

Mulvey, G. (2013) *In Search of Normality: Refugee Integration in Scotland*. Glasgow: Scottish Refugee Council.

Papadopoulos, R.K., Rashid Y.M. and Mahamed, Z. (2010) *Enhancing Vulnerable Asylum Seekers Protection (EVASP), UK National Report*. UK: Centre for Trauma, Asylum and Refugees (CTAR), University of Essex.

UNODC (UN Office on Drugs and Crime) (2012) *Global Report on Trafficking in Persons*. Vienna: UNODC.

Wren, K. (2007) 'Supporting asylum seekers and refugees in Glasgow: the role of multi-agency networks', *Journal of Refugee Studies*, 3: 391–413.

World Health Organization (2013) *Humanitarian Health Action: Migrant Health*. Geneva: WHO.

Zimmerman, C., Kiss, L. and Hossain, M. (2011) 'Migration and health: a framework for 21st century policy-making', *PLoS Medicine*, 85(5).

PRIMARY HEALTHCARE

MERLIN WILLCOX, BRIAN D. NICHOLSON AND DAVID MANT

Chapter overview

After reading this chapter you will be able to:

- explain what primary care is and the services it delivers
- explain why primary care is essential to the delivery of MDGs for health
- identify the main barriers to the delivery of effective primary care
- evaluate solutions to overcome delivery barriers.

INTRODUCTION

Primary health care (PHC) is the first point of contact with a health worker, usually in a community health centre relatively near to the patient's home. Its role is to diagnose and treat most simple diseases, recognize and refer in cases of any serious illnesses and offer preventive interventions, such as family planning, antenatal care and vaccinations. In contrast, 'secondary' care is delivered in hospitals, often further from the patient's home and the main focus is curative care and treatment of more serious or unusual illnesses that require admission to hospital, surgery or input from a specialist. 'Tertiary' care refers to specialized hospitals that provide a service to the whole region or country for the treatment of conditions needing more specialized services, such as heart surgery or organ transplantation.

PHC is important to all healthcare systems because, without it, health outcomes are worse and cost-efficiency is reduced. As the healthcare system in the USA demonstrates, trying to deliver healthcare without effective primary care leads to very high costs that are unaffordable for most countries. Moreover, this high level of expenditure does not achieve better (and sometimes achieves demonstrably worse) health outcomes for the individual. Thus, PHC is a central feature of all national healthcare systems delivering high-quality affordable universal care (Starfield, 1994). In cost-efficient health systems, PHC 'coordinates care when people receive services at other levels of care' (Starfield, 2008). Although Starfield's evidence derives from HICs in Europe and North America, her findings apply also to LMICs. The importance of PHC is almost certainly inversely proportional to the size of the health budget (Figure 8.1, Starfield, 2002). The less that is available to spend on health, the more important it is to prevent and treat effectively in low-cost ambulatory settings.

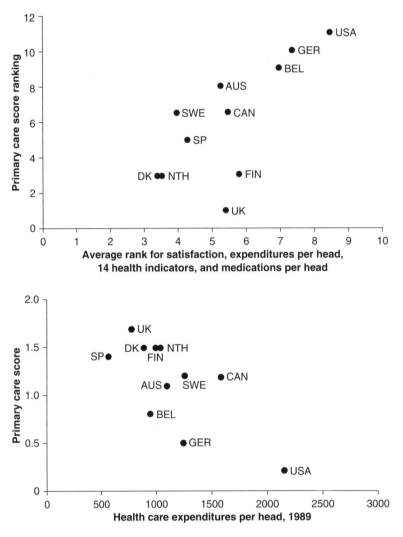

Figure 8.1   The relationship between healthcare costs and outcomes in 11 countries

Source: Starfield (2002), reproduced by permission of Elsevier.

The International Conference on Primary Healthcare in Alma-Ata (then the USSR, now Kazakhstan) in 1978 produced the famous Alma-Ata Declaration and goal of health for all by the year 2000 (HFA2000). It defined PHC as, 'the first element of a continuing healthcare process', which delivers 'essential healthcare based on practical, scientifically sound and socially acceptable methods and technology made universally accessible to individuals and families in the community through their full participation and at a cost that the community and country can afford to maintain at every stage of their development in the spirit of self-reliance and self-determination.'

Activity 8.1

Google HFA2000 and list the main elements of the PHC approach.

Comment

Key elements of PHC described in the Alma-Ata Declaration were:

- education concerning prevailing health problems and the methods of preventing and controlling them
- promotion of food supply and proper nutrition
- an adequate supply of safe water and basic sanitation
- maternal and child healthcare, including family planning
- immunization against the major infectious diseases
- prevention and control of locally endemic diseases
- appropriate treatment of common diseases and injuries
- provision of essential drugs.

The World Health Organization (WHO) has reaffirmed its commitment to the Alma-Ata approach. Emphasizing the importance of delivering care locally without requiring people to travel long distances, the WHO (2008) stresses the value of community development, teamwork, patient-centred care, good local governance and empowerment of people to take responsibility for their own health. Although these underlying principles help to set aims and objectives, they do not show how to overcome the barriers that have blocked their implementation over the past 35 years. Some of these barriers reflect necessary trade-offs between different objectives, such as local devolution often leading to inequity of provision and quality.

The obvious barrier to implementation of the objectives enshrined in the Alma-Ata Declaration in LMICs is lack of resources. Countries with similar levels of resources, however, vary substantially in their success in delivering adequate quality PHC. Some countries seem to manage universal delivery of the key PHC services necessary to reach MDG targets (vaccination; nutrition and hygiene support; safe maternity services; effective first contact acute care for serious disease) with relatively little, while others with more resources fail. Success seems to depend on overcoming three common operational issues:

- inadequate human resources to staff PHC, evidenced by limited ability to recruit and retain high-quality staff, particularly in disadvantaged areas
- poor leadership, public regard and professional status
- lack of public and clinical governance of performance.

Failure to deliver effectively the PHC services that reduce health system costs (prevention and care of chronic diseases; effective diagnosis and prioritization for hospital referral) leads to a vicious cycle of health system failure. The health system becomes less efficient and demand for costly hospital care increases, further reducing the resources available to fund the PHC services that can control costs (see Chapter 2). The rest of this chapter therefore focuses on the practical issue of how to implement and deliver high-quality PHC cost-effectively.

HOW TO DELIVER PHC

The eight elements of PHC identified as important in 1978 fail to spell out in adequate detail four key functions that PHC must provide in order to improve health outcomes while allowing governments to provide universal healthcare for an affordable cost. These are:

- preventive care, such as vaccinations, antenatal care and measuring blood pressure
- effective diagnosis and care of acute illness to prevent progression of disease, such as the early treatment of malaria, bacterial chest infection and acute diarrhoea
- management of long-term conditions (LTCs), as all but the most acute phases of LTCs can be managed effectively outside hospital
- diagnostic triage for serious illness and control of hospital referral, as most acute illness can also be managed effectively in the community.

The Alma-Ata Declaration stressed the importance of intersectoral collaboration with agencies outside the health services. Two of the four functions – preventive care and the provision of care for people with serious LTCs after hospital discharge (such as those with untreatable or terminal illnesses) – obviously require effective intersectoral liaison as well as community involvement and empowerment. In fact, all four functions require close liaison within the health sector – with hospital specialists and other disciplines. A key role for PHC, therefore, is coordinating care across health sectors.

PRACTITIONERS OF PHC

Effective multidisciplinary teamwork and local ownership are common features of successful systems. An example of the successful implementation of such an approach on a large scale is the Brazil Family Health Programme.

The key challenge for this large and diverse country was to achieve its Millennium Development Goal (MDG) health targets, such as reducing the infant mortality rate. Introducing a multidisciplinary PHC team system with a strong community focus enabled it to achieve this. It successfully promoted key public health interventions (such as feeding practises and vaccinations) and improved the management of common childhood infections so that, adjusting for changes in other health determinants, the infant mortality rate fell by 4.5 per cent for every 10 per cent step increase in population coverage (Macinko et al., 2006).

A number of strategies have been shown to enhance PHC teamwork. Multiskilling and task shifting allow the available team members to be deployed efficiently. The optimal composition of the PHC team, however, will depend not only on local service priorities but also the local availability and competence of individual staff groups.

There is substantial international literature that highlights the potential for role substitution, particularly nurses taking on roles traditionally performed by doctors (Laurant et al., 2005). There is some evidence, too, that training voluntary community health workers can be effective in improving the delivery of PHC (Brenner et al., 2011). Although there has been much controversy surrounding the training of traditional birth attendants (TBAs), clear evidence exists that effective training programmes can reduce perinatal mortality (Wilson et al., 2011). The programmes that were most effective were embedded in a wider health system intervention. Training TBAs, it seems, only works as part of an horizontal approach, not as a single vertical programme (Bhutta et al., 2011).

A key challenge in many countries is not just a shortage of health workers but also the fact that most health workers do not want to work in PHC for reasons of low pay, status, inadequate support, inadequate facilities and the disadvantages of working in a rural location (Moosa et al., 2013). Competitive salaries work, but non-monetary incentives, such as the provision of autonomy, plus good working and living conditions are also effective – as, in the longer term, is prioritizing recruitment of trainees from those living in underserved areas (Sundararaman and Gupta, 2011; see Chapter 3). The introduction of specialist training (with accreditation and mandatory continuing professional medical education (CME) and appraisal) is also an essential step in developing a medical workforce with the necessary knowledge and skills to provide an adequate quality of PHC.

In most LMICs, doctors are hardly ever found in PHC settings. Instead, nurses and midwives are often expected to treat patients (although their formal training seldom includes this skill) and often even they are unavailable, especially in remote rural clinics. Then, the only healthcare providers may be healthcare assistants with little or no formal training. The immediate priority must therefore be to train and support these workers. The evidence suggests strongly that ongoing support and supervision is more important than one-off training. Information technology (IT) can make this possible (Were et al., 2013).

Activity 8.2

You have just been appointed as district medical officer and find that none of the rural health centres in your district has been able to recruit a doctor to work there.

1. List the likely causes.
2. What local action would you take to manage this situation?
3. What action could be taken by regional or central government?

Comment

An inability to appoint staff to PHC facilities is a common problem. It can be mitigated by the actions at both local and national level discussed in this chapter and Chapter 3. Some of these actions increase the likelihood of recruitment, while others mitigate the problem by implementing role substitution teamwork and changes in the skills mix.

The difficulty with staffing doctor posts in rural PHC settings has led to calls to move away from the UK concept of doctor-led teams. This makes sense, although effective diagnostic triage (gatekeeping) requires high-level clinical skills and the ability to both assess and manage risk – skills that doctors are specifically trained to undertake. It is also crucial that the referral system (so people can move from one level to the next) works effectively.

ACCESSING PHC

The delivery of PHC depends on access, so it should be delivered as near to the patients as possible, which also increases the likelihood of effective community involvement. There is clearly a trade-off to be made, however, as you cannot have a fully staffed health centre in every village – it would be neither affordable nor possible to staff it.

The evolution of health systems into primary, secondary and tertiary tiers reflects the need to make such trade-offs, but these tiers describe functions, not necessarily facilities. It is possible, and sometimes necessary, for a single health facility to deliver more than one tier of service. It may be operationally better for PHC to be delivered locally (by peripatetic village-based health workers), but managed more centrally, from a secondary or even tertiary care facility. A number of vertical programmes (such as HIV/AIDS, TB and malaria control outreach programmes) have demonstrated the effectiveness of this approach.

The rapid development of technology – both IT and medical equipment – affords new possibilities for the delivery of care. Mobile phone coverage has become almost universal in many countries, even LMICs. Diagnostic technology has become smaller, cheaper, more robust and more mobile, so it can be used in PHC settings. Diagnostic technology linked to the Internet and mobile phone networks harness both central expertise and facilitate self-care, making it possible to:

- support PHC workers at a distance
- provide PHC workers with much better tools for diagnostic triage
- support patients self-caring for LTCs through mobile phone links.

A number of initially very successful community-based PHC systems in LMICs (such as Brazil) have, unfortunately, found themselves under pressure when the basic needs have been met and there is an increase in demand for higher standards of care. Almost all countries (LIC or HIC) are experiencing increasing demand for high-technology care. Even in the UK, an increasing number of people each year bypass local PHC facilities and present directly to secondary care, meaning it must be geared-up to provide a cost-efficient PHC service. One possible solution is to increase the availability of diagnostic technology in primary care so hospital attendance is unnecessary to access it. Technological advances mean that diagnostic testing can now sometimes be done as reliably and more cost-effectively in primary care than in hospital with appropriate quality assurance.

HOW TO ORGANIZE AND GOVERN PHC

This section considers issues of funding, modes of delivery and how quality is assured.

FUNDING PHC

Healthcare can be financed through direct payment by those who attend, some form of voluntary or compulsory insurance, or taxation. Government policy determines whether staff are independent contractors or employees and if health worker payment is linked to performance through capitation, fee for service or pay for performance mechanisms, all of which can work really well or really badly, depending on how well they are implemented. Formal analysis has reiterated this point – the funding system does not predict the quality of the care (Starfield, 2008). Choosing a system that is feasible to implement locally is a key determinant of its success or failure.

Research shows that user fees stop the most impoverished groups from accessing care, but removing fees may have unintended consequences and actually reduce the quality of the care if it impacts significantly the funding available for the service (Lagarde and Palmer, 2011). For example, UNICEF's Bamako Initiative in 1987 tried to improve the availability of medicines by charging 'user fees' (Garner, 1989). This worked, but it also increased irrational prescribing and reduced access for the poorest people (Uzochukwu et al., 2002). In response, Uganda has abolished user fees, but without any commensurate increase in public funding, so public services are overstretched and lack essential medicines.

Caution is always necessary when applying evidence from other countries and generalizing from high-income to low-income settings, but it is clear that governments do not necessarily have to employ staff directly in order to provide a publically funded PHC service. For example, the taxation-funded NHS in the UK provides universal access to PHC by commissioning care from multidisciplinary clinical teams led by general practitioners working as independent for-profit contractors.

Activity 8.3

Visit the Cochrane Collaboration's website and find the evidence base for the effectiveness of financial incentives in promoting quality care.

Comment

> A substantial body of evidence has examined the different options for financing and delivering PHC in different countries, although the best solution depends strongly on local context. It is less a matter of what system works best and more about whether the conditions that make a particular solution work well exist in the relevant country. Two Cochrane reviews – one focusing on PHC (Scott, et al., 2011) one focusing on PHC (Scott et al. 2011), one on studies in LICs (Witter et al., 2012) – highlight the need for caution and customization when applying the evidence to other settings.

SHOULD PHC BE ORGANIZED AS DISEASE-SPECIFIC VERTICAL PROGRAMMES?

One of the key principles of PHC is that it deals with whatever problems people present. Even in high-income settings, patients often lack the knowledge and support to self-diagnose and assign themselves to appropriate disease-specific 'vertical' care. Also, many patients have more than one medical problem at any one time.

Some aspects of PHC can be delivered very effectively through centrally organized disease-specific 'vertical' programmes targeting diseases such as HIV/AIDS, TB, polio and malaria. The success of a vertical approach usually reflects a high level of external funding, but it may well also reflect a strong focus on training and support for health workers, plus strong central systems of governance.

Governance of vertical programmes is easier because they are implementing 'evidence-based', cost-effective interventions for a range of illnesses, often with clear quality performance indicators. For example, one review identified 16 evidence-based interventions that, if implemented, could reduce neonatal mortality by over 50 per cent (Darmstadt et al., 2005). In many HICs, most key preventive services, such as vaccinations and cancer screening, are organized as centrally run vertical programmes, even if they are delivered in PHC facilities.

If there were vertical programmes for every cost-effective intervention, however, this could:

- drive up costs, because staff are scarce
- fracture continuity of care, as people often have more than one problem
- compromise equity as, for example, palliative care drugs available for patients with terminal HIV are not for those with terminal cancer and drug cupboards full of antiretrovirals have no anti-malarials
- fail to engage successfully with local communities, as delivering appropriate and effective care very often depends on the ability to understand the local culture and circumstances of the individual.

----------------------------------- Activity 8.4 -----------------------------------

List reasons for community involvement being important. Identify risks posed by decentralization.

Comment

The Alma-Ata Declaration stresses the importance of community involvement, which appears important for meeting MDGs. Decentralization can lead to substantial local variations in the quality of care, however. PHC programmes that require the application of modern technology and strong quality assurance may be more effective if they are governed centrally.

The key challenge is therefore to bring together the strengths of both horizontal and vertical approaches to delivering PHC. This is not easy. The solution in the UK, of focusing the vertical programmes on preventive care and integrating them within PHC, has already been adopted in some LMICs, but seldom in government-funded facilities. This is usually because of gross disparities in resources (which create inequity and disrupt salary structures) and organizational rigidity on the part of both NGOs and government departments.

The following box shows the outcome of a Cochrane review that explored the evidence regarding the benefits of integrating specific vertical programmes into 'horizontal' PHC provision.

What is the evidence?

The effects of integrating vertical programmes into PHC

A Cochrane review (Dudley and Garner, 2011) assessing the effects of strategies to integrate PHC services on healthcare delivery and health status in LMICs concluded:

> There is some evidence that 'adding on' services (or linkages) may improve the utilization and outputs of healthcare delivery. However, there is no evidence to date that a fuller form of integration improves healthcare delivery or health status. Available evidence suggests that full integration probably decreases the knowledge and utilization of specific services and may not result in any improvements in health status. More rigorous studies of different strategies to promote integration over a wider range of services and settings are needed. These studies should include economic evaluation and the views of clients, as clients' views will influence the uptake of integration strategies at the point of delivery and the effectiveness on community health of these strategies.

This Cochrane review indicates that the integration of vertical and horizontal programmes is feasible, but is often implemented unsuccessfully. This failure to integrate is detrimental to the health system. Those responsible for 'horizontal' PHC services must recognize the benefits that external resources, staff training and good governance can bring. Both NGOs and government agencies responsible for vertical programmes need to recognize that the patients' usual PHC workers are best placed to assess their needs and coordinate the delivery of interventions, taking into account the priorities and social context of the community they serve and their patients' other health priorities.

ASSURING QUALITY

A common weakness of PHC is geographical variation in care quality. Quality is often inversely correlated to need – the 'inverse care law' (Vitoria, 2008).

Poor-quality services, wastage, corruption and weak management still characterize many community-based PHC institutions in India, with considerable variations in care both within and between states. A particular problem in some rural PHC centres are absentee workers ('ghosts'), with up to a 50 per cent absentee rate reported at spot checks in some areas (Das and Hammer, 2007). Similar 'absentee worker' rates have been reported in sub-Saharan Africa, usually associated with inadequate or unpaid wages and the consequent need to take on more than one job. Absenteeism is a form of fraud and the reported experiences of PHC workers from sub-Saharan Africa suggest that, in many places, the remoteness and decentralization of PHC facilitate such corruption (Moosa et al., 2013).

Africa carries 25 per cent of the global burden of disease, but only has 3 per cent of the world's health workers (WHO, 2006). Within Africa, most of the health workers are concentrated in relatively affluent urban areas and a similar study of PHC staffing in India characterized the situation as, 'Not enough here ... too many there' (WHO, 2006). Remote rural areas, which have the greatest need, have the greatest shortage of health workers (Moosa et al., 2013).

Problems of recruiting and retaining high-quality staff to work in PHC, particularly in disadvantaged areas, have been discussed. The quality of the medical staff in PHC is often particularly poor. For example, a 2007 World Bank investigation of healthcare in Delhi reported that doctors in PHC centres were less competent and made less effort than staff in the hospital sector, particularly the private hospital sector (cited in WHO, 2007: 42).

Probably the most important solution to this cause of differential care quality is to ensure that there is no negative differential in pay or clinical facilities for health workers working in PHC, particularly in disadvantaged areas. That does not eliminate the need to continually assess care outcomes against evidence-based national and international standards, however.

In the UK, governance of general practice is achieved partly by creating a demand-led situation – giving patients choice as to which PHC providers they register with, so they can 'vote with their feet'.

National standards are applied and implemented in five other ways:

- quality-assuring training and exit examinations, including professional specialist accreditation
- continuing professional training with annual appraisal and (for doctors) five-yearly assessment of continued fitness to practice through revalidation (relicensing)
- clinical performance assessment against evidence-based quality standards – both process outcomes (such as quality of prescribing) and outcome measures (such as proportion of diabetic patients with HbA1c levels below 7 per cent)
- auditing and investigations of adverse outcomes (such as the national confidential enquiries into maternal and child deaths) and the annual audit of public satisfaction with the services offered at each PHC facility.

PHC teams in the UK enjoy substantial organizational and professional freedom, provided their performance in these five areas meets national standards.

The authors were involved in a quality improvement programme in Uganda and Mali based on the auditing and investigation of adverse outcomes. The case study below happened in south-west Uganda in 2013. It flags up some failures in clinical care, but also the way in which PHC provision is complicated by sociocultural factors, which need to be understood and, indeed, are more likely to be recognized, not missed, by well-trained PHC teams.

The key factor in the success of this approach in PHC is the participation of all stakeholders (including the community and healthcare providers) in the discussion of deaths, how they could have been avoided and formulating and implementing solutions.

Case study   From a death review in Uganda, October 2013

A six-month-old baby girl fell ill with a mild cough, cold and runny nose. The next morning, she developed a fever and her grandmother took her to a private clinic, where they consulted an enrolled nurse. She did a malaria test, which was positive, prescribed zinc sulphate and paracetamol and advised taking the child to hospital. The grandmother, instead, decided to take the child to a traditional healer, who performed some traditional cleansing rituals. The child remained ill with a high fever and intermittent diarrhoea until she passed away the same night.

The function of PHC is fulfilled by many more actors than just the qualified health workers in the official clinics. Patients initially may choose to visit:

- pharmacists, owners of chemists
- traditional or complementary therapists
- priests and faith healers (Bodeker and Burford, 2007).

To improve care, all may need to participate. Investigating what went wrong is a powerful mechanism for improving healthcare, but people will not participate (or will not tell the truth) if they feel they will be blamed. 'Confidential enquiry' is a methodology that identifies and disseminates key lessons without assigning blame to individuals. The above example illustrates that these lessons are often complex, requiring action at a community as well as health facility level.

The ongoing assessment of clinical performance in the UK is made possible because recording of all clinical activity undertaken in PHC facilities, including prescribing and recording of medical records, is now electronic – as is the linked financial management system. The rapidly decreasing cost of IT and the leading role of many MICs in IT innovation, means that implementing such systems to support clinical governance and quality assurance could be cost-effective for many health systems. If it is only possible to have a paper-based system, it is important to restrict duplicate data collection to the minimum – time spent filling in forms that are not important for the ongoing care of the patient diverts health workers from providing care and can reduce its quality.

The other key factor increasing the ability to monitor the quality of PHC is patient registration. Although this effectively reduces consumer choice, it clarifies who is responsible for providing care to a defined population and provides a firm denominator for measuring performance. This is particularly important when measuring the quality of preventive activities, such as screening and vaccinations.

One of the simplest and potentially most effective governance strategies is to focus on the availability and appropriate use of a small number of low-cost generic drugs known to be effective for the major causes of mortality and morbidity. The availability of cheap, effective generic drugs, manufactured in MICs, such as India, is increasing and should help deliver high-quality cost-effective PHC. There is a substantial and helpful body of literature on successful strategies to improve the quality of prescribing in LIC settings (Ayieko et al., 2011).

QUALITY NOT QUANTITY

The WHO points to the absolute lack of trained PHC workers in most LMICs, but increasing their numbers does not necessarily help. Government pressure to increase numbers when there is a shortage of skilled workers often leads to the recruitment of poorly motivated, unskilled individuals who undermine the motivated workers in their provision of high-quality care. It is almost certainly a better strategy to dismiss the substandard workers and pay the best workers twice as much to cover the extra work. Identifying who is delivering poor-quality care depends on setting and monitoring quality standards.

CONCLUSION

PHC is the patient's first point of contact with a health worker, although its scope extends beyond clinically trained professionals to a range of social and support workers. It is crucial to have robust systems in place to train, support and regulate the health workers who actually provide care, whatever their professional status. The skills mix, role substitution and teamwork all have to be facilitated and professional restrictions dismantled if PHC is to work well and help address the existing unequal access to healthcare that exists within and between countries. Universal coverage implies pooling financial risk through either direct taxation or insurance and this is in place in many countries, but monitoring, audit and review (clinical governance) are also essential to assure quality.

REFERENCES

Ayieko, P., Ntoburi, S., Wagai, J., Opondo, C., Opiyon, N., Migrio, S. et al. (2011) 'A multifaceted intervention to implement guidelines and improve admission paediatric care in Kenyan district hospitals: a cluster randomised trial', *PLoS Medicine* 8(4): e1001018.

Bhutta, Z.A., Soofi, S., Cousens, S., Mohammad, S., Memon, Z.A., Ali, I. et al. (2011) 'Improvement of perinatal and newborn care in rural Pakistan through community-based strategies: a cluster-randomised effectiveness trial', *The Lancet*, 377: 403–412.

Bodeker, G. and Burford, G. (eds) (2007) *Public Health & Policy Perspectives on Traditional, Complementary & Alternative Medicine.* London: Imperial College Press.

Brenner, J.L., Kabakyenga, J., Kyomuhangi, T., Wotton, K.A., Pim, C., Ntaro, M. et al. (2011) 'Can volunteer community health workers decrease child morbidity and mortality in southwestern Uganda? An impact evaluation', *PLoS ONE,* 6: e27997.

Darmstadt, G.L., Bhutta, Z.A., Cousens, S., Adam, T., Walker, N. and De Bernis, L. (2005) 'Evidence-based, cost-effective interventions: how many newborn babies can we save?' *The Lancet,* 365: 977–988.

Das, J. and Hammer, J. (2007) 'Money for nothing: the dire straits of medical practice in Delhi, India', *J Dev Econ,* 83: 1–36.

Dudley, L. and Garner, P. (2011) 'Strategies for integrating primary health services in low- and middle-income countries at the point of delivery', *Cochrane Database Syst Rev*, CD003318.

Garner, P. (1989) 'The Bamako initiative', *BMJ*, 299: 277–278.

International Conference on Primary Healthcare (1978) *Declaration of Alma-Ata* [Online]. Alma-Ata, USSR. Available at: www.who.int/publications/almaata_declaration_en.pdf (accessed 18 July 2012).

Lagarde, M. and Palmer, N. (2011) 'The impact of user fees on access to health services in low- and middle-income countries', *Cochrane Database Syst Rev,* 13(4): CD009094.

Laurant, M., Reeves, D., Hermans, B., Braspenning, J., Grol, R. and Sibbald, B. (2005) 'Substitution of doctors by nurses in primary care', *Cochrane Database Syst Rev*, 18(2): CD001271.

Macinko, J., Guanais, F.C., De Fatima, M. and De Souza, M. (2006) 'Evaluation of the impact of the Family Health Program on infant mortality in Brazil, 1990–2002', *J Epidemiology Community Health,* 60(1): 13–9.

Moosa, S., Wojczewski, S., Hoffmann, K., Poppe, A., Nkomazana, O., Peersman, W. et al. (2013) 'Why there is an inverse primary-care law in Africa', *The Lancet Global Health,* 1: e332–e333.

Starfield, B. (1994) 'Is primary care essential?', *The Lancet,* 344(8930): 1129–33.

Starfield, S. and Shi, L. (2002) 'Policy relevant determinants of health: an international perspective' *Health Policy*, 60(3): 201–18.

Starfield, B. (2008) 'The future of primary care: refocusing the system', *N Engl J Med*, 359(20): 2087–2091.

Sundararaman, T. and Gupta, G. (2011) 'Indian approaches to retaining skilled health workers in rural areas', *Bull World Health Organ*, 89(1): 73–77.

Uzochukwu, B.S., Onwujekwe, O.E. and Akpala, C.O. (2002) 'Effect of the Bamako-Initiative drug revolving fund on availability and rational use of essential drugs in primary healthcare facilities in south-east Nigeria', *Health Policy and Planning*, 17: 378–383.

Vitoria, C.G. (2008) 'The millennium development goals and the inverse care law: no progress where it is most needed?', *J Epidemiol Community Health*, 62(11): 938–939.

Were, M., Nyandiko, W., Huang, K., Slaven, J., Shen, C., Tierney, W. et al. (2013) 'Computer-generated reminders and quality of pediatric HIV care in a resource-limited setting', *Pediatrics* 131(3): e789–96.

Wilson, A., Gallos, I.D., Plana, N., Lissauer, D., Khan, K.S., Zamora, J. et al. (2011) 'Effectiveness of strategies incorporating training and support of traditional birth attendants on perinatal and maternal mortality: meta-analysis', *BMJ*, 343: d7102.

World Health Organization (2006) *World Health Report: Working Together for Health.* Geneva: WHO.

World Health Organization (2007) *WHO Country Office for India. Not Enough Here, Too Many There: Health Workforce in India.* Geneva: WHO.

World Health Organization (2008) *The World Health Report. Primary Healthcare: Now More than Ever.* Geneva: WHO.

COMMUNICABLE DISEASES

COLIN S. BROWN AND WILLIAM NEWSHOLME

Chapter overview

After reading this chapter you will be able to:

- describe the burden of infectious diseases
- explain how disease burden is used and the limitations of data
- describe programmes for control of communicable diseases.

INTRODUCTION

Though there are various ways in which to measure disease burden, no matter what metric is used, communicable diseases continue to wreak havoc on the young and working-age populations in LMICs. Furthermore, communicable diseases disproportionately affect the poor.

MEASURES OF DISEASE BURDEN

Disability-adjusted life years (DALYs) is a widely used metric to describe disease burden. Infectious diseases account for a significant proportion of DALYs. The Global Burden of Disease Report suggested that lower respiratory tract infections, diarrhoeal illnesses, human immunodeficiency virus (HIV) and acquired immunodeficiency syndrome (AIDS), malaria and tuberculosis (TB) accounted for approximately one fifth of global morbidity in 2004 (Murray et al., 2012). Updates in 2010 revised these estimates downwards (see Table 9.1 for longitudinal trends), in keeping with the increased dual burden of infectious and non-communicable diseases the global South now faces. Rapid increases in cardiovascular disease, diabetes and mental illness are coupled with sustained lost DALYs from infectious diseases (Murray et al., 2012).

Global mortality is dominated by the same five infectious processes, which were responsible for 8 (15 per cent) of the estimated 53 million deaths in 2010 (Lozano et al., 2012), though case fatality rates for most infections have fallen since 1990. For absolute numbers, some 2,000,000,000 have been infected at some point with the hepatitis B virus, with roughly the same number latently infected with TB.

Media attention is focused on new and emerging pathogens with pandemic potential (severe acute respiratory syndrome (SARS), H7N1 influenza) and those that catch the attention of the tabloids, such as *Naegleria fowleri*, the 'brain-eating amoeba'. Viral haemorrhagic fevers have always captured the public imagination, even before the devastating West African outbreak of the Ebola virus disease in 2014 (Dye, 2015).

Table 9.1   Global burden of disease estimates for the top five communicable diseases, 2000–2010

Top five communicable diseases*	2000**	2004**	2010***
Lower respiratory tract infections	6.4	6.2	4.6
Diarrhoeal illnesses	4.2	4.8	3.6
HIV/AIDS	6.1	3.3	3.3
Malaria	2.7	2.2	3.3
Tuberculosis	2.4	2.2	2.0
Totals	21.8	18.7	16.8

Key

* Percentages of global DALYs

** WHO, Global Burden of Disease studies

*** Institute for Health Metrics and Evaluation

CHALLENGES

While much progress has been made in the fight against many of the major communicable diseases (HIV/AIDS, TB and malaria), there is still far to go. The emerging challenge of antimicrobial resistance (AMR), leading to multi-drug resistant (MDR) strains, modern animal husbandry increasing the potential for zoonotic spread and changes in priorities for research and development all exemplify the ever-changing landscape of disease control. Mass population movement, urbanization and globalization affect the speed and diversity of infection transmission. Environmental change, alterations in agricultural land use and changes in vector populations due to trade and climate change also increase the potential for the spread of infectious diseases.

This chapter describes programmes that have effectively reduced disease transmission and been successfully implemented globally. The lesser-known neglected tropical diseases (NTDs), under-represented by DALY measurement due to limitations in current surveillance, and measurement of how being a chronic carrier affects morbidity is also covered (Mathers et al., 2007). A snapshot is provided of some of the global health challenges of infectious disease control, but the chapter does not review important childhood diseases (see Chapter 13), including acute respiratory infections, diarrhoeal diseases or vaccine-preventable diseases. Insight into the challenges faced by practitioners in a globalized world is provided where international travel, changing patient demographics, diagnostic and treatment challenges and international security concerns are increasingly ubiquitous.

Activity 9.1

List reasons for measuring disease burden and some problems with doing so.

Comment

Comparing burdens helps with strategic health planning, enabling the prioritization and provision of health services. Also, treatment costs can be estimated and how the disease burden is likely to change under various policies and interventions can be assessed. Think about the limited availability of data on long-term morbidity, particularly for neglected diseases, which have not received much political attention or treatment research and development. There are also concerns about methodology, such as disability and age weighting in DALYs, lack of good descriptive epidemiology and data collection bias.

TB AND HIV/AIDS

GLOBAL BURDEN

TB and HIV/AIDS are the largest infectious killers of adolescents and working age groups, taking over from diarrhoeal and respiratory illness seen in neonates and childhood. By 2010, HIV/AIDS, TB and injuries combined were responsible for over half of all deaths of 20- to 39-year-old men (Lozano et al., 2012).

The Joint United Nations Programme on HIV/AIDS (UNAIDS) estimated that by 2012 there were some 34 million people living with HIV or AIDS (PLWHA) worldwide. Though total numbers of new infections are falling, having declined by 20 per cent over the past decade, there were still around 2.5 million new cases in 2011 (UN, 2012). With a widespread scaling up of antiretroviral therapy (ART) provision, global mortality has fallen by one quarter since 2005, though there were still around 1.7 million deaths in 2011. There remain wide geographical disparities. For example, decreases in new cases seen in sub-Saharan Africa (approximately 70 per cent of all living cases/global mortality occur in sub-Saharan Africa) have been mirrored by increases in North Africa, Eastern Europe and the Middle East.

Approximately a third of the world's population is infected with TB, with 5 to 10 per cent of these becoming infectious or ill at some point. In 2011, an estimated 8.7 million people were newly infected, with 1.4 million deaths, of whom 430,000 were HIV co-infected. Some 80 per cent of the world's TB burden is concentrated in 22 countries, with more than half of cases in just five (India, China, Pakistan, Bangladesh and Indonesia). Encouragingly, TB mortality has sharply dropped since 1990 – by some 41 per cent by 2011 – and concurrently there has been a steady decline in incident cases. Drug-resistant strains threaten to challenge this decline (WHO, 2012a).

INTERNATIONAL TARGETS

The Millennium Development Goals (MDGs), adopted by the UN in 2000, set bold targets for global poverty reduction, with Goal 6 ('Combat HIV/AIDS, malaria and other diseases') mandating that, by 2010, there would be universal access to treatment for HIV/AIDS and, by 2015, a reversal in the spread of HIV/AIDS (UN, 2013). Unfortunately, by 2011, seven million people still lacked access to ART. Further goals were set by UNAIDS to revolutionize HIV prevention and care by 2015 and achieve the ultimate – 'Getting to zero' (UN, 2010).

- **Zero new infections** Halving sexual transmission and eliminating vertical and intravenous transmission.
- **Zero AIDS-related deaths** Enabling universal access to ART, halving TB-related and AIDS-related maternal mortality and making social support available.
- **Zero discrimination** Halving number of countries with punitive laws and travel or residency restrictions and zero tolerance for gender-based violence, with all countries delivering social protection strategies and at least half specifically addressing the needs of women.

Implementation of interventions intended to limit the spread of TB were 'far below targets set in the Global Plan in 2006' (WHO, 2008b). By 2015, these ambitious goals aimed for all PLWHA to be screened for TB and, if diagnosed, commenced on ART (WHO, 2006). By 2012, fewer than 50 per cent of those co-infected received ART (UN, 2012). Though the global TB programmes look on track to achieve the MDG goal of a 50 per cent mortality reduction by 2015 (WHO, 2012a), the 50 per cent target for PLWHA is unlikely to be reached.

INTERVENTIONS

The WHO's efforts to control TB are based on the concept of directly observed therapy, short course (DOTS), which aims to detect and treat infectious cases and so reduce transmission and the spread of drug resistance. DOTS programmes are comprised of five elements: diagnosis, observed therapy, treatment monitoring, short-course therapy with guaranteed drug supplies and government commitment to sustainability. The WHO's Global Plan to Stop TB (WHO, 2006) has six components:

1. Pursue high-quality DOTS expansion and enhancement.
2. Address TB-HIV, MDR-TB and the needs of poor and vulnerable populations.
3. Contribute to health system strengthening based on primary health care.
4. Engage all care providers.
5. Empower people with TB and communities through partnership.
6. Enable and promote research.

Constraints to putting disease control into practice arise from outdated diagnostics that are difficult to utilize in resource-constrained settings, the latency and chronicity of disease, as well as the length of treatment, hampering the diagnosis and management of cases, plus a lack of infrastructure and staff.

HIV/AIDS programmes need to address similar problems, aiming to stop transmission through sexual health measures, slow progression by early diagnosis and treatment and reduce or eliminate vertical and nosocomial transmission. As for TB, diagnosis and laboratory monitoring can be difficult, but a modified DOTS programme, DOT-HAART, is one model of care that is proving useful (Farmer et al., 2001).

TREATMENT GUIDELINES

Initiating HIV treatment early slows progression of the disease (Franco and Saag, 2013) and may prevent transmission. Mathematical modelling suggests that an immediate and sustained reduction in HIV incidence could be achieved in South Africa using this approach (Granich et al., 2009), though caution has been voiced regarding the feasibility of this in resource-limited settings, where universal treatment may not be available (Wagner and Blower, 2012). Others have questioned its adoption in any setting, citing limited evidence of population or individual benefit (Cambiano et al., 2011: Lundgren et al., 2013). In June 2013, the WHO changed its ART treatment initiation recommendations to 500 CD4 cells/µL. The UK, awaiting the results of the strategic timing of antiretroviral treatment (START) study, expected in 2016, has not changed its guidelines (ClinicalTrials.gov, 2009).

Scaling up poses significant challenges to countries already struggling with the treatment costs associated with the recent changes to treatment guidelines, with the threshold altering from 200 to 350 CD4 cells/µL in 2010 (WHO, 2013c). It has been suggested that there will be, 'profound cost implications on Global Fund, PEPFAR and developing country health budgets' and that, 'expecting countries to move to a costly new CD4 threshold without sufficient evidence is a mistake' (Geffen, 2013). Both TB and HIV programmes must simplify, decentralize and task shift to allow them to access at risk populations sustainably.

INTEGRATION OF TB/HIV SERVICES

One reason for a dual focus on HIV and TB is the synergistic ability of TB to take advantage of the cell-mediated immunity deficiencies caused by HIV (Murray, 1990). Additionally, TB:

- progresses faster in PLWHA
- is harder to diagnose in PLWHA
- in PLWHA, is almost certain to be fatal if undiagnosed or left untreated
- occurs earlier in the course of HIV infection than many other opportunistic infections.

By 2012, only 40 per cent of all TB patients had a documented HIV test result (WHO, 2012a). In vertical single-disease programmes, staff may be unaware of the complex interactions between the two disease processes or may be unable to address them appropriately, which is why it is important to harmonize services (Lipman and Breen, 2006) and integrate TB and HIV disease control strategies.

A variety of integration models exist, such as the Médecins Sans Frontières' (MSF) South African model of complete integration in a 'one-stop shop' (Kerschberger et al., 2012). Integrated service delivery models, in areas suffering an undue burden of dual infection (mainly Sub-Saharan Africa), offer significant benefits to patients who 'often [have] to navigate complex health systems to secure access', allowing for 'care integrated within one facility' that 'should serve patients best (with caveats around TB infection control) and promote efficient use of resources (Legido-Quigley et al., 2013).

DRUG RESISTANCE

Drug resistance affects both TB and HIV, arising from primary infection with resistant strains, poor adherence to therapy or inadequate access to quality-controlled drugs. Laboratory constraints make monitoring for resistance difficult in LMICs, both before and during treatment.

Multi-drug resistant tuberculosis (MDR-TB), where the mycobacteria has resistance to the two most important antimycobacterials, is increasing. In 2011, over 60,000 cases were identified worldwide, the majority in India and China (WHO, 2012a). Lack of TB antimicrobial culture and drug susceptibility testing in many countries suggest this figure underestimates the reality. Worldwide, 3.7 per cent of new cases and 20 per cent of previously treated cases were estimated to have MDR-TB (WHO, 2012a). More recently, extensively drug resistant TB (XDR-TB) has been recognized (Gandhi et al., 2006), posing a serious threat to global TB control because treatment options are then limited to more toxic drugs with limited efficacy.

To combat these threats, the WHO, in association with the Stop TB Partnership, set up the Green Light Committee Initiative to provide countries with access to high-quality, second-line drugs. Despite this, the spectre of totally drug resistant TB (TDR-TB) has become reality (Udwadia et al., 2012). New drug development is therefore an urgent priority.

Bedaquiline, the first novel class of antimicrobial agent for TB in 40 years, was approved by the US Food and Drug Administration in December 2012 for drug resistant TB (WHO, 2013b). As Table 9.2 illustrates, most drugs routinely used for TB were discovered over half a century ago. The perceived lack of markets in developed countries is cited as a cause of the lack of ongoing investment.

Table 9.2 Antituberculous drug development

Mainstay TB chemotherapeutics	Year developed
Isoniazid*	1952
Pyrazinamide	1954
Ethambutol	1962
Rifampicin*	1963
Moxifloxacin	1999

(Continued)

Table 9.2   (Continued)

MDR-/XDR-TB chemotherapeutics	
Streptomycin	1944
PAS	1948
Prothionamide	1951
Cycloserine	1955

* Resistance to both = MDR-TB

Activity 9.2

Discuss with colleagues why funding for HIV therapeutics greatly exceeds that for TB. Think of reasons for a country preferring to keep its HIV and TB control programmes separate.

Comment

The large numbers of men initially infected with HIV in the West received prominent media attention early in the epidemic and campaign groups such as Treatment Action Group in the USA and Treatment Action Campaign in South Africa mean that a powerful lobby for funding persists, with access to cheap therapeutics and funding (human resources, health systems and programme grants for treatment) through agencies such as the Global Fund to Fight AIDS, TB and Malaria. Apart from reticence by funders and providers who have vested interests in keeping pathways separate, the cross-transmission of TB to HIV patients is a concern.

MALARIA

GLOBAL BURDEN

Malaria is endemic in 109 countries, with 3.3 billion at risk of infection and it killed approximately 660,000 people in 2010, with a global estimate of 219 million cases. The overwhelming disease burden is in sub-Saharan Africa, with 50 per cent of all cases occurring in four countries (Nigeria, Democratic Republic of Congo, Kenya and Tanzania).

Thanks to current interventions, 274 million cases and 1.1 million deaths have been averted since 2000, with approximately half of these being in the top ten high-burden countries (WHO, 2012b).

While historically a major cause of infectious disease mortality, there is also increasing evidence for its significant morbidity, including premature birth and growth retardation, chronic anaemia, undernutrition and neurological sequelae impacting schooling, as well as the risk of contracting HIV due to the need for blood transfusions.

The accuracy of disease estimates in south Asia is being questioned (Dhingra et al., 2010).

INTERNATIONAL TARGETS

The cornerstones of malaria control are infection prevention through the use of insecticide-treated bed nets, indoor residual spraying and intermittent prophylaxis; diagnosis using classical microscopy or rapid dipstick tests; treatment with artemisinin-containing compounds; and surveillance and systems building. The four-point Roll Back Malaria control plan mandates the following key areas of work (WHO, 2010a):

- prompt access to treatment, ensuring all infected (particularly children) receive effective medication
- insecticide-treated bed nets (ITNs), with the main challenge to scale up their use
- prevention and control of malaria in pregnant women, as they are particularly susceptible to anaemia, perinatal mortality and low birthweight babies
- malaria epidemic and emergency responses, to help prevent mortality in those populations with little or no exposure to malaria.

The targets endorsed by the World Health Assembly in 1998 call for a 75 per cent reduction in malaria cases by 2015 on the levels in 2000 (WHO, 2011). The WHO's oversight of the programme has recently been restructured into the Global Malaria Programme, advised by the Malaria Policy Advisory Committee, and a new 'Test, treat, track' model is being introduced (WHO, 2012c).

DRUG AVAILABILITY AND MISUSE

The ability of health services to implement these control elements is constrained by being unable to provide accurate diagnostics using either classical blood microscopy or rapid antigen–antibody dipstick tests and difficulty in maintaining drug supplies.

Syndromic management, using protocols such as the WHO's Integrated Management of Childhood Illness (WHO, 2005) and novel drug supply chain innovations, such as 'ColaLife', may be some of the systems available to tackle these difficulties (Coca-Cola, 2011). Other methodologies include intermittent preventive therapy (IPT), which is when populations in endemic areas are treated during the seasonal months to interrupt transmission, whether infected or not. The positive effect of reductions in malaria incidence and mortality need to be weighed against the possible threat of developing drug resistance. Some argue that overdiagnosis and potential mismanagement of other causes of febrile illness negate the utility of syndromic treatment (Perkins and Bell, 2008) and rapid, cheap, sensitive diagnostics are the way forward. Those who favour IPT point to its cost-effectiveness (Carneiro et al., 2010).

Drug resistance to many of the classical anti-malarials is increasing and the use of newer artemisinin-based compounds may already be under threat, with reports of resistance in the Thai–Cambodia border (Yeung et al., 2009). Widespread use of counterfeit medicine is also of concern. One large review found that of approximately 4000 samples from South East Asia and sub-Saharan Africa, 35 per cent failed chemical analysis, though it was unclear how much was due to manufacturing failure or nefarious marketing (Nayyar et al., 2012).

ERADICATION VERSUS ELIMINATION

Two terms used incorrectly and interchangeably in common parlance are:

- **eradication** the global, permanent removal of a disease from the Earth by removal of the pathogen
- **elimination** the global reduction of the prevalence of a disease to a negligible level or complete removal of it from a certain area of the world, without removal of the pathogen.

The Bill & Melinda Gates Foundation has put financial and political weight behind malaria eradication (Bill & Melinda Gates Foundation, 2013). There has, however, been considerable debate about whether the global community should instead aim for elimination from some countries and control in highly endemic regions (Tanner and de Savigny, 2008). Marked reduction has been achieved in malaria transmission using current control methods in some of the borderline endemic areas (Feachem et al., 2010).

CLIMATE CHANGE AND INSECTICIDE USE

Warmer summer temperatures in previously mosquito-free climes threaten the global targets for elimination. In countries that have not seen endemic malaria in recent memory, migrant workers and returning travellers pose a health risk as their febrile illness, if undiagnosed, may lead to new propagation due to changing mosquito habitats, as seen in Greece in 2012 (Sudre et al., 2013). Changes in mosquito range in tropical countries is also extending transmission areas (WHO, 2010b).

Current mosquito control methods using insecticide-treated bed nets and indoor residual spraying also are threatened, by both the possibility of environmental effects and the development of mosquitoes' resistance to available insecticides.

─────────────────── **Activity 9.3** ───────────────────

List the major problems facing malaria control.

Comment

You may have thought about competing needs for scarce resources. Fake drugs, political instability, lack of cheap interventions that will limit disease and threats to drug and insecticide effectiveness due to unregulated use in medicine and agriculture are other possibilities.

Resources intensively invested into widespread and expensive eradication programmes may remove the spectre of malaria from the world, but you may believe this is impossible and so elimination is a more cost-effective measure that can hope to contain the disease indefinitely at negligible levels. Similar discussions are prevalent around polio and, more recently, measles.

ANTIMICROBIAL RESISTANCE

GLOBAL BURDEN

Antimicrobial resistance (AMR) has been recognized as a problem in the global North for years. There are few global estimates of AMR, though it is indeed a global problem. Meticillin-resistant *Staphylococcus aureus* (MRSA) and resistance in gram-positive organisms has long been a focus of attention, but there are increasing worries about resistance in gram-negative organisms. New Delhi metallo-beta-lactamase-1 (NDM1), a mutation resistant to carbapenem antibiotics, emerged in India and has removed from many settings the last mainstay of broad-spectrum antimicrobial therapy as organisms containing this mutation are frequently pan-resistant to all but two antibiotics (polymyxin and tigecycline). It can easily jump between environmental and human *Enterobacteriaceae* through plasmid-transfer and was identified in nearly every continent within a year of its discovery. International air travel facilitated its rapid dissemination (Molton et al., 2013).

Typhoid has also seen increases in resistance to widely used antibiotics, such as chloramphenicol, ampicillin and trimethoprim-sulfamethoxazole (Zaki and Karande, 2011). Resistance to the mainstays of treatment of MDR typhoid fever, ceftriaxone and ciprofloxacin, are now rising, too (Nath and Maurya, 2010). Increased antimicrobial stewardship, surveillance and infection control measures are thus a global concern (Molton et al., 2013). The 2011 UK Chief Medical Officer's report mentions that, without antimicrobials, 'modern surgery would be unacceptably dangerous' and 'cancer chemotherapy and organ transplantation … would no longer be viable' (Davies, 2012).

DRUG AVAILABILITY AND MISUSE

In many LMICs, certain classes of medicine regulated in high-income settings (such as TB medication) are freely available to be prescribed by private practitioners removed from the state health infrastructure, many of whom use inappropriate and expensive regimes (Uplekar and Rangan, 1993). In addition, drugs can be purchased from pharmacies without the need to obtain a prescription from qualified healthcare providers (Net, 2012). For diseases such as TB, which need prolonged, uninterrupted treatment, a failure in the supply chain and infrastructure can cause serious consequences for global disease control and individual outcomes. Paul Farmer (2003) has eloquently argued that the intermittent supply of TB drugs seen in Russian prisons is a serious form of human rights abuse.

ANIMAL TO HUMAN TRANSMISSION

No matter how much attention is paid to antimicrobial control in humans, globally, the vast majority of drugs used are in the veterinary setting, given mainly to prevent illness among animals farmed intensively.

Animal to human transmission of AMR, either through direct consumption or run-off into local water supplies, demands global attention and has been called 'an ecological tragedy akin to the tragedy of the commons' (Conloy, 2010). The complex interaction of antimicrobials used in veterinary and plant agriculture settings, as well as the 'introduction of antimicrobial compounds into the aquatic environment via medical therapy, agriculture, animal husbandry and companion animals', has allowed for an environment, particularly in waste water collections, in which the proliferation of AMR in resident environmental bacteria can become rife (Cantas et al., 2013).

These examples highlight why national approaches must exist within a broader context of international monitoring and control of disease.

--- Activity 9.4 ---

List who needs to be engaged in talks about measures to control AMR.

Comment

This is a global problem, requiring the consensus, attention and multidisciplinary approach of 'medical doctors, dentists, veterinarians, scientists, funders, industry, [and] regulators', as well as international monitoring and control through changes in prescribing practices and 'drug licensing, financial incentives, penalties, and ban or restriction on use of certain drugs' (Cantas et al., 2013).

NEGLECTED TROPICAL DISEASES (NTDS)

GLOBAL BURDEN OF DISEASE

The term 'neglected tropical diseases' (NTDs) was coined in 2005, following recognition that there is gross international neglect of many conditions that cause tremendous amounts of global disease burden.

There is no accepted definition of NTDs, however, with several different agencies defining the scope in different ways. The WHO's current list of NTDs is shown in Table 9.3. In general, they can be thought of as diseases of the marginalized poor, confined to the tropics and tending to cause morbidity and disability rather than mortality. The NTDs have been neglected over the years by both local health systems and the international drug development and research communities for a variety of reasons (Kappagoda and Ioannidis, 2012).

One Global Burden of Disease (GBD) review counted African trypanosomiasis, Chagas disease, schistosomiasis, leishmaniasis, lymphatic filariasis, onchocerciasis, intestinal nematode infections, Japanese encephalitis, dengue, and leprosy, calculating that, in 2002, they accounted for approximately 177,000 deaths worldwide, mostly in sub-Saharan Africa, and about 20 million DALYs, which is 1.3 per cent of the global burden of disease and injuries (Mathers et al., 2007). The WHO estimates suggest over one billion people are affected by at least one NTD, but it is not

Table 9.3   Types of NTDs

Chronic bacterial infections
Buruli ulcer
Leprosy
Trachoma
Yaws

Insect-borne
African and South American trypanosomiasis
Dengue
Leishmaniasis
Lymphatic filariasis
Onchocerciasis

Soil-transmitted helminths
Ascaris
Hookworm
Strongyloides
Trichuris

Water source/sanitation-related helminths
Schistosomiasis
Guinea worm
Hydatid

Food-related helminths
Cysticercosis
Fasciola

Others
Podoconiosis
Rabies
Snakebite

uncommon for an individual to be co-infected with several pathogens, particularly in the case of the helminths. Some have postulated that the poor outcomes seen in treating TB and other conditions in sub-Saharan Africa, compared to contemporary or historical counterparts, may be due to the high burden of parasitic infection borne in the region, with exaggerated host responses to disease and poor response to vaccination (Li and Zhou, 2013).

Because of the large disability burden, it can be argued that DALYs lost due to infection provide a better estimate of disease burden (see Table 9.4). DALYs themselves are problematic disease measures, particularly when used for decisionmaking and resource allocation, for reasons such as argument over weighting values, problems of uneven disease clustering in populations and failure to account for the impact of the disease on families reliant on the affected individual (Anand and Hanson, 1997).

Table 9.4   Estimation of DALYs attributed to NTDs

Disease	DALYs	Infected globally
Hookworm	22.1 million	576 million
Ascaris	10.5 million	807 million
Trichuris	6.4 million	604 million
Lymphatic filariasis	5.8 million	120 million
Schistosomiasis	4.5 million	207 million
Trachoma	2.3 million	84 million
Onchocerciasis	0.5 million	37 million
Totals	52.1 million	> 1 billion

Source: Fenwick (2012)

Mathematical modelling suggests the enormous impact of these diseases, such as estimating the annual costs as seven billion US dollars for South American trypanosomiasis (Lee et al., 2013).

Complex problems associated with the breakdown of health systems in post-conflict areas have also led to outbreaks of NTDs, such as African trypanosomiasis following periods of violence in the Democratic Republic of Congo (Lutumba et al., 2005).

ERADICATION AND ELIMINATION

In 1965, the world's first global disease programme to eradicate a specific pathogen celebrated its success as smallpox disappeared from the world (with two remaining samples held within government laboratories in the USA and Russia). Other pathogens followed, with polio within its sights. Though polio control efforts remain well funded, the future of its eradication is threatened by lack of progress within four countries (India, Pakistan, Afghanistan and Nigeria). This prompted calls for whether or not such high levels of funding should be sustained, given that they could be invested in other health programmes (Barrett, 2009). Guinea worm is the only NTD for which there is a near-completed eradication programme. Total funding for NTDs reflects only about 0.6 per cent of international development investment, with recent examples of disinvestment.

Historically, leprosy has carried stigma. Each year, over 100,000 new cases are identified and, although elimination is a global target (and was broadly achieved in 2000), concerns over local increases in several settings have been raised, with some calling for clarification around definitions of control and elimination targets and concerns over incorrect initial incidence estimates and large numbers of cases being found by active surveillance. The possibility of drug resistant strains is also of concern, as free provision of combination drug therapy from Novartis through the WHO is currently only guaranteed until 2015 (Dogra et al., 2013). Such donations provide a great percentage of NTD treatment. For example, between 2008 and 2012, an estimated 3.39 billion albendazole tablets were donated by GlaxoSmithKline and 1.97 billion ivermectin tablets by Merck (Hotez et al., 2009).

DISEASE CONTROL

Current control programmes for other NTDs are based on five key areas of intervention.

1. **Preventive chemotherapy** Valid for schistosomiasis and helminths, reducing morbidity and decreasing transmission. As an additional benefit, it may kill other infections not directly targeted. For example, one dose of invermectin, albendazole and praziquantil is curative for schistosomiasis, but also will treat onchocerciasis and lymphatic filariasis (Anto et al., 2011). Such measures can provide a platform for other public health interventions, such as vaccination programmes, and allow for the potential of community medication distributors, such as teachers.
2. **Intensified case management** Useful for trypanosomiasis and leishmaniasis, where the key difficulty is early diagnosis and then treating and managing complications effectively. This needs a robust healthcare system and so exemplifies how improving PHC across all settings will lead to robust improvements in population health (Walley et al., 2008).
3. **Vector control** Many NTDs have insect vectors, so there is a pressing need to better understand vector biology, as well as use large quantities of good-quality pesticides, address environmental concerns and prevent the development of resistance. The misuse of pesticides in agriculture and the more recent release of genetically modified insects pose concerns for future disease control (Matthews et al., 2011; Reeves et al., 2012).
4. **Provision of safe water, sanitation and hygiene** Some 800 million people lack access to safe drinking water, while 2.5 billion lack sanitation, with ongoing problems of both provision and maintenance of supply, particularly in sub-Saharan Africa where NTDs are rife (United Nations Children's Fund, 2012).
5. **Veterinary public health** Several of the NTDs have links with agriculture or wild animals. For instance, the life cycle of African trypanosomiasis involves cattle and herd movement as a source of outbreaks. Thus, effective animal health is key to stopping transmission.

All have potential challenges, many of which relate to the alleviation of poverty; the possibility of reinfection following treatment; population growth and migration, urbanization; the movement of livestock and vectors; changes in land usage; and climate change.

Activity 9.5

Discuss with colleagues who influences the priority setting for the Global Burden of Disease (GBD)?

Comment

You may have thought of the pharmaceutical industry, specialist charities, NGOs and academic research groups. Did you also consider the effect of political expediency? Many NTDs (though not all) arise from the underlying determinants of health – poverty, access to food and clean water, basic sanitation and overcrowding. The political will to combat these basic conditions could be championed by climate change and human rights advocates, as well as politicians, bolstered by public support for basic access to rights.

HEALTHCARE-ASSOCIATED INFECTION (HCAI)

For some years now, the impact and control of healthcare-associated infection (HCAI) has received much attention in HICs. The incidence of HCAI is between 4 and 7 per cent in these settings, with an incidence of surgical site infection approaching 3 per cent. Excess costs from HCAI have been estimated at $4.5 billion in the USA and up to a third of these infections are entirely avoidable. There is also good evidence that relatively simple interventions can significantly reduce infection rates (Haley et al., 1985).

Until relatively recently, however, data from LMICs has been lacking. Some data from Mexico and Trinidad from the mid-1990s considered estimated mortality rates and cost (Orrett et al., 1998; Ponce-de-Leon, 1991), but only when two major studies were published in 2011 did the true impact begin to emerge.

What is the evidence?

Allegranzi et al. (2011) showed, in published data from resource-poor countries from 1995 to 2008, a pooled HCAI prevalence of:

- 15.5/100 patients
- an incidence of HCAI in adult Intensive Care Unit (ITU) of 47.9/1000 patient days
- an incidence of surgical site infection of 5.6/100 procedures.

Similar work by Bagheri et al. (2011), looking specifically at data from sub-Saharan Africa, showed a pooled HCAI prevalence of:

- 2.5 to14.8 per cent
- an incidence HCAI of 5.7 to 48.5 per cent
- an incidence of surgical site infection of 2.5 to 30.9/100 procedures (up to 83 per cent in some dirty procedures).

Though many studies are of low quality, this suggests that, compared to HICs, hospitalwide, the incidence of HCAI is two to three times that in the global North, surgical site infections are up to 20 times more common, infection rates in critical care are up to 13 times and, in neonatal units, up to 20 times those seen in HICs.

In HICs, relatively simple, sustainable interventions, such as establishing a specific infection control practitioner in a hospital, supervising infection control committees and the use of simple guidelines, significantly reduce infection rates (Atif et al., 2006; Danchaivijitr et al., 1996; Hodges and Agaba, 1997).

The impact of HCAI has been acknowledged at a global level at the World Health Assembly in 2002. The 2008 WHO Africa region conference resulted in health ministers from 26 African countries committing to improvement programmes. Leading on from this, the WHO launched the Global Patient Safety Challenge, using a series of two- to three-year cycles to identify and target key issues. Areas already addressed are 'Clean care is safe care', focusing on simple hand hygiene interventions, a surgical safety checklist (SSCL) and a safe childbirth check-list (WHO, 2013a), for which increasingly good evidence exists as to their efficacy (Allegranzi et al., 2011; Haynes et al., 2009).

Effective intervention remains hampered by a lack of funding, lack of national policy or plans, low use of existing guidelines, such as the WHO's SSCL, poor stocks of equipment and alcohol-based hand hygiene rubs, weak training both pre- and in-service and a lack of point-of-care reminders in the workplace.

Activity 9.6

Identify some challenges facing LMICs regarding nosocomial infections.

Comment

Some ideas you may have thought of include few or no operating procedures for cohorting infectious patients. Here, patients infected or colonized with the same infectious agent are put together, confining care to one area and preventing contact with other susceptible patients. Microbiological capacity for identifying drug-resistant strains and assessing transmission within hospitals is limited. Managerial responsibility for patient safety within care settings is lacking, too. Also, problems with ventilation and heating that do not allow for adequate protective precautions and lack of consistent access to personal protective equipment for staff are constraints.

INTERNATIONAL HEALTH MONITORING

Before 2003, coronaviruses were thought to cause 'common colds', an upper res-piratory and gastrointestinal tract virus, in mammals and birds. The only two known circulating strains then (now five) caused mild, self-limiting symptoms. In 2003, SARS emerged – a fatal new coronavirus that originated in East Asia, with 8096 cases and 774 deaths worldwide (WHO, 2004). Concerns over lack of international reporting of SARS were raised: 'WHO member states [had] no international legal obligation ... to report SARS cases to WHO or to refrain from certain trade and travel-restricting measures aimed at stopping the spread of SARS' (Fidler, 2003).

Thus, in an increasingly globalized, interdependent world, a consensus has been formed that nations can no longer operate solely within their own boundaries. Rather, their responsibility for health protection extends to their neighbour states and beyond. The International Health Regulations (IHR) were rewritten taking this new political reality into account. They were codified in 2005 by the WHO and the UN and were built on existing work that originated from the International Sanitary Regulations in 1969. There was a limited number of reportable diseases (initially six, then three – cholera, plague, and yellow fever) and the approach to the spread of dis-ease internationally was not coordinated (WHO, 2007). These regulations place strict requirements on countries, so, when a threat emerges within their borders, they must inform the relevant authorities, including the WHO, the European Centre for Disease Prevention and Control (ECDC) in Europe and other relevant agencies, as well as having the core capacity to surveil and control communicable diseases. Global infor-mation sharing has also become prominent, through WHO alerts and the Harvard-run Programme for Monitoring Emerging Diseases – ProMED (Woodall, 1997).

A subsequent, novel coronavirus was identified in London in September 2012, again causing pulmonary and renal failure (Assiri et al., 2013). This was the second case in the world – the first case having been diagnosed and reported through Pro MED in Saudi Arabia the previous week and then swiftly reported under the IHR to all relevant authorities and named Middle East respiratory syndrome coronavirus (MERS-CoV).

The diagnosis of this second individual – a Qatari national who had recently visited Saudi Arabia and travelled to London for tertiary-level care – was prompted by the ProMED report (Bermingham et al., 2012). Thus, his clinical samples were tested for genetic material common to all coronaviruses. Global collaboration has since identified the possible reservoir of the virus as a bat widespread in the Middle East (Memish et al., 2013).

Real-time surveillance is being increasingly used globally. Each year, Public Health England (which took over from the Health Protection Agency and the National Treatment Agency for Substance Misuse), diagnoses the onset of influenza through syndromic surveillance, whereby sentinel sites of general practice report increases in flu-like symptoms. This precedes laboratory diagnosis by some two weeks and tweets of flu-like symptoms have been shown to pre-empt disease activity and 'offer the potential to crowdsource epidemics in real time' (Collier et al., 2011). In advance of the Olympic Games in 2012, communicable disease surveillance was increased to include unexplained respiratory illness in ITU settings (that is, its aim was to identify MERS-like disease; Severi et al., 2012).

CONCLUSION

This chapter has introduced key concepts in global communicable disease surveillance and control. Funding interests, political expediency, conflicting priorities, increasing resistance patterns (often fuelled by poor prescribing), interdependence of global practice and the reshaping of international migration – all contribute to the changing face of disease control.

An interdisciplinary global health response is required to face these challenges. Basic science researchers, clinical and public health practitioners, politicians, social scientists, economists, geographers, historians and other disciplines must collaborate to learn from past and present success and failures in disease prevention and control.

FURTHER INFORMATION

Public Health England www.gov.uk/government/organisations/public-health-england

NathNAC www.nathnac.org

ISARIC isaric.tghn.org

WHO www.who.int

Global Fund to Fight AIDS, Tuberculosis and Malaria www.theglobalfund.org

Joint United Nations Programme on HIV/AIDS www.unaids.org

Bill & Melinda Gates Foundation www.gatesfoundation.org

REFERENCES

Allegranzi, B., Bagheri Nejad, S., Combescure, C. et al. (2011) 'Burden of endemic health-care-associated infection in developing countries: systematic review and meta-analysis', *The Lancet*, 377: 228–241.

Bagheri, N., Allegranzi, B., Syed, S.B. et al. (2011) 'Health-care-associated infection in Africa: a systematic review', *Bull World Health Organ*, 89: 757–765.

Cantas, L., Shah, S.Q., Cavaco, L.M., Manaia, C., Walsh, F., Popowska, M. et al. (2013) 'A brief multi-disciplinary review on antimicrobial resistance in medicine and its linkage to the global environmental microbiota', *Front Microbiol*, 4: 96.

Feachem, R.G., Phillips, A.A., Hwang, J., Cotter, C., Wielgosz, B., Greenwood, B.M. et al. (2010) 'Shrinking the malaria map: progress and prospects', *The Lancet*, 376: 1566–1578.

Fenwick, A. (2012) 'The global burden of neglected tropical diseases', *Public Health*, 126: 233–236.

Granich, R.M., Gilks, C.F., Dye, C., De Cock, K.M. and Williams, B.G. (2009) 'Universal voluntary HIV testing with immediate antiretroviral therapy as a strategy for elimination of HIV transmission: a mathematical model', *The Lancet*, 373: 48–57.

Mathers, C.D., Ezzati, M. and Lopez, A.D. (2007) 'Measuring the burden of neglected tropical diseases: the global burden of disease framework', *PLoS Negl Trop Dis*, 1: e114.

Murray, C.J., Vos, T., Lozano, R., Naghavi, M., Flaxman, A.D., Michaud, C. et al. (2012) 'Disability-adjusted life years (DALYs) for 291 diseases and injuries in 21 regions, 1990–2010: a systematic analysis for the Global Burden of Disease Study 2010', *The Lancet*, 380: 2197–2223.

UN (2010) *Getting to Zero: 2011–2015 Strategy Joint United Nations Programme on HIV/AIDS (UNAIDS)*. Geneva: UNAIDS.

WHO (2007) *International Health Regulations*, 2nd edition. Geneva: World Health Organization.

WHO (2012c) *Test. Track. Treat. Scaling Up Diagnostic Testing, Treatment and Surveillance For Malaria*. Geneva: WHO.

WHO (2013c) *WHO Issues New HIV Recommendations Calling for Earlier Treatment* [Online]. Geneva: WHO. Available at: www.who.int/mediacentre/news/releases/2013/new_hiv_recommendations_20130630/en/ (accessed 23 January 2015).

A complete list of references is available at: https://bugsanddrugs.wordpress.com/gh/book-references/

10

NON-COMMUNICABLE DISEASES, INJURIES, SUICIDE AND SELF-HARM

RHYS WILLIAMS AND ANN JOHN

Chapter overview

After reading this chapter you will be able to:

- define the terms 'non-communicable diseases', 'injuries', 'suicide' and 'self-harm'
- identify the extent to which these contribute to the global burden of disease
- explain the degree to which they are preventable and the evidence base supporting this
- outline public health strategies and other global initiatives relevant to the management and prevention of these conditions and how we should 'think globally and act locally'.

INTRODUCTION

This chapter deals with the increase in the incidence, prevalence and impact, in virtually all countries of the world, of the major non-communicable diseases (cardiovascular disease, chronic lung disease, the major cancers and type 2 diabetes), the increasing individual and public health burden following injuries of all types and the devastating effects of suicide and other forms of self-harm. Mental health, of crucial importance for understanding suicide and self-harm, is addressed in Chapter 11.

The importance to public health of the conditions dealt with here has several facets:

- three out of five deaths are caused by these conditions
- long-term disability results, reducing the quality of life for millions of people
- they impact negatively on national economies because of lost productivity

- they impose a massive burden on national health and social care systems, as well as on individuals and families
- there is potential for prevention through modifying the social environment to reduce known risk.

Despite the WHO's recognition of the importance of these conditions, global funding for development assistance for health (DAH) remains skewed towards communicable rather than non-communicable diseases. Although this position has improved since Nugent and Feigl (2010) reported that under 3 per cent of DAH was devoted to the latter, improvement has been slight.

FROM 'DISEASES OF AFFLUENCE' TO THE 'TRIPLE WHAMMY'

When European-trained physicians and surgeons first started working in sub-Saharan African countries, the pattern of disease they encountered was totally different from that which they had left behind in Europe. In the 1940s and 1950s, appendicitis, constipation and diverticular disease were the most common gastro-enterological conditions among European patients. Coronary heart disease and type 2 diabetes were rare and largely confined to the more affluent members of society. The predominant cancers were those of the stomach, colon and breast, with lung cancer becoming more common year on year, particularly in men. These conditions were virtually unknown in the patients encountered in sub-Saharan Africa.

Over time, this epidemiological pattern changed in both Europe and sub-Saharan Africa. In Europe, diseases such as coronary heart disease and type 2 diabetes ceased to be associated mostly with affluence and became conditions affecting all sections of society. Now they are more frequent in the comparatively poor.

In Africa, as diets and other factors changed with Westernization and increasing urbanization, common European afflictions of constipation, appendicitis and diverticular disease became more frequent. Later, the common European cancers and coronary heart disease, type 2 diabetes and stroke emerged. Initially, the sectors of African society most affected were the relatively affluent.

The situation today is that most sectors of society in LMICs are prone to these formerly 'European' non-communicable diseases. They no longer affect largely the economically well off either. They have joined the communicable diseases that formerly dominated the disease patterns of sub-Saharan Africa and other similar countries (and still provide daunting public health challenges) and, together with an epidemic of injury (largely the result of violence, occupational hazards, self-harm and road traffic incidents), are the components of what has been termed the 'triple whammy' now hitting LMICs worldwide.

─────────────────── Activity 10.1 ───────────────────

Enter the search term 'non-communicable diseases' on the WHO's website (at: www.who. int/en). Read the most recent factsheet on this subject. Pay particular attention to the 'WHO response' section regarding this global health challenge. Access and study one of the WHO's strategic documents mentioned under that heading.

THE CONTRIBUTION OF THESE CONDITIONS TO THE CURRENT GLOBAL BURDEN OF DISEASE

An extensive international multi-agency effort has quantified the extent of the burden that different diseases and disease categories impose on individual countries, regions and the world as a whole. This Global Burden of Disease study produced estimates for 1990, 2005 and 2010 using comparable measures so that time trends and comparisons between diseases and between countries and regions may be studied in a valid way. The measures used in this study are years of life lost (YLLs), years lived with disabilities (YLDs) and disability-adjusted life years (DALYs).

YLLs are the number of years of life lost for each disease or group of diseases, taking account of mortality from the disease and the number of years of life expectancy lost as a result of this mortality. The calculation of YLDs uses the prevalence of various forms of disability from each disease, weighted by the severity of each disability. DALYs are the sum, for each disease or group of diseases, of YLLs plus YLDs. DALYs are thus a composite measure of the burden of any disease, in terms of both its effect on premature mortality and its effect on disability.

Between 1990 and 2010, an important shift was noted between the contributions of DALYs resulting from the broad groups of diseases shown in Table 10.1.

Table 10.1   Shift in the distribution of DALYs worldwide from 1990 to 2010

	DALYs (worldwide total and proportion of the total)	
Disease group	1990	2010
Communicable, maternal, neonatal and nutritional disorders	1.18 billion 47 per cent	0.87 billion 35 per cent
Non-communicable diseases	1.08 billion 43 per cent	1.34 billion 54 per cent
Injuries	0.24 billion 10 per cent	0.28 billion 11 per cent
Total (all conditions)	2.50 billion	2.49 billion

Source: Adapted from Murray et al. (2012)

Although the world's disease burden had decreased slightly, the burden of non-communicable diseases had increased, both in absolute terms and as a proportion of the whole, while there was a reduction in communicable, maternal, neonatal and nutritional disorders, with the contribution of injuries staying much the same. In 2010, the most important single cause of death and disability worldwide was ischaemic heart disease (in 1990 it had been the fourth most important), followed by lower levels for respiratory infections (it had been top in 1990). HIV/AIDS had moved rank from thirty-third in 1990 to fifth in 2010.

The contribution in DALYs of the top 20 conditions in 2010 are shown in Table 9.2, together with the rankings for those same conditions in 1990. The conditions that are discussed in this chapter have asterisks by them.

Table 10.2 The top 20 conditions (in terms of DALYs) in 2010 and their previous rankings in 1990 in the Global Burden of Disease study

Rank in 2010	Disease or condition	No. of DALYs (worldwide) in 2010	Rank in 1990
1	Ischaemic heart disease*	129,820	4
2	Lower respiratory infections	115,227	1
3	Stroke*	102,232	5
4	Diarrhoea	89,513	2
5	HIV/AIDS	81,547	33
6	Lower back pain	83,063	11
7	Malaria	82,685	7
8	Preterm birth complications	76,982	3
9	Chronic obstructive pulmonary disease (COPD)*	76,731	6
10	Road injury*	75,482	12
11	Major depressive disorder	63,179	15
12	Neonatal encephalopathy	50,150	10
13	Tuberculosis	49,396	8
14	Diabetes*	46,823	21
15	Iron-deficiency anaemia	45,338	14
16	Neonatal sepsis	44,236	17
17	Congenital anomalies	38,887	13
18	Self-harm*	36,654	19
19	Falls*	35,385	22
20	Protein–energy malnutrition	34,874	9

Source: Adapted from Tables 1 and 5 in Murray et al. (2012)

The six conditions highlighted (ischaemic heart disease, stroke, COPD, road injury, diabetes (types 1 and 2 combined), self-harm and falls) contribute just under 40 per cent of the total DALYs consequential to these top 20 conditions.

No specific cancer sites are included in these top 20 conditions, though neo-plasms as a whole contributed 188,487 DALYs (7.5 per cent of the 2010 total). Within the overall category of neoplasms, those of the trachea, bronchus and lung are by far the largest contributor (32,405 DALYs), with those of the liver second (19,111), followed by those of the stomach (16,413), colon and rectum (14,422) and breast (12,018).

Although, in HICs, many initiatives are directed at better clinical management, early detection through screening and primary prevention of several cancers, pro-gress has been much less marked in LMICs. Among the reasons for this are a lack of surveillance infrastructure, such as cancer registries, lack of effective screening programmes for cervical and breast cancer and the general lack of healthcare resources. As Buonaguro et al. (2013) commented, 'there is a dearth of information about the burden, pathogenesis, and therapeutic approaches about cancer in resource-limited countries'.

Activity 10.2

From what you already know of the risk factors and preventive and therapeutic measures for the diseases and conditions listed in Table 10.2, identify likely reasons for the changes in the rankings for 1990 and 2010. Pay particular attention to those rising significantly in relative importance and those that have fallen.

Comment

Since this is a 'league table' of the impact of conditions relative to each other, individual conditions may change in their rankings even though their absolute impact in terms of DALYs may not. Indeed, it is possible for the absolute impact of any condition to increase (or decrease) and for them to fall (or rise) relative to others.

Conditions that have risen in both absolute and relative terms include ischaemic heart disease and diabetes (largely the result of an increase in type 2 diabetes) and HIV/AIDS. The increases seen in the first two of these are the result of complex changes in lifestyle in relation to diet and physical activity and possibly increased awareness of the conditions among healthcare professionals and the general public.

The rise in HIV/AIDS is consequent on person-to-person transmission by means of unsafe sexual practices and the sharing of needles among intravenous drug users (see Chapter 9).

The absolute and relative fall in the impact of diarrhoea (particularly diarrhoea in childhood) is the result, among other factors, of the provision of clean water and effective sanitation, the promotion of breastfeeding and safe and effective methods for rehydration in those affected (see Chapter 13).

For TB, important factors have been the identification and effective treatment of cases and their contacts (often with 'directly observed' therapies), the screening of at risk populations and the organized use of BCG vaccination (see Chapter 9).

ECONOMIC IMPACT

The major non-communicable diseases have an impact that can be measured not only in terms of the YLLs and YLDs but also in terms of their effect on the economy. Days of work lost through illness and the premature mortality and disability of economically active members of the workforce can be estimated by the 'human capital' approach. This equates the value of a unit of lost production to the wages or salary that society would have paid for the work to be done. This approach has been criticized as overestimating the value of that work since, in reality, unemployed members of society are usually recruited into the workforce to replace those lost to the workforce through death or disability.

Any such overestimation by the human capital approach, however, is more than compensated for by the failure to factor in the lost productivity when unpaid but nevertheless essential work is left undone – when, for example, those responsible for running households or caring for children are unable to do so because of premature mortality or the onset of disability. Estimates such as those given in Table 10.3 are thus likely to be underestimates of economic growth lost as a result of heart disease, stroke and diabetes in nine individual countries. The WHO (2005) describes this economic impact as 'unappreciated'.

What is the evidence?

Table 10.3   Projected national income forgone due to heart disease, stroke and diabetes over the ten years from 2005 to 2015 in nine selected countries

Countries	Lost income (international dollars*)	Countries	Lost income (international dollars*)
Brazil	45 billion	Pakistan	35 billion
Canada	10 billion	Russian Federation	300 billion
China	558 billion	United Kingdom	40 billion
India	220 billion	United Republic of Tanzania	5 billion
Nigeria	10 billion		

* The 'international dollar' is a currency measure that corrects for the different purchasing power of the US dollar in different countries.

Source: WHO (2005)

The economic impact of these conditions on individuals and families depends on the health and social care systems in the countries where they live. Where universal healthcare coverage exists, the economic impact at the point of delivery of care will be zero or close to zero, the funding for the care having been derived from direct taxation. In countries where universal healthcare coverage is not the norm, the cost to the family and the individual may be considerable and the effect on family life and well-being can be devastating. Uninsured and underinsured individuals may forgo treatment altogether or have to settle for inadequate treatment.

Worldwide, suicide is the thirteenth leading cause of death for people of all ages, but it is one of the three leading causes of death among those in the most economically productive age group (15–44 years), the other two being road traffic injuries and interpersonal violence. This prominence among existing and future economically active members of society means that suicide has a disproportionately high impact on national economies that is over and above what would be expected for the numbers of deaths involved if taken alone.

ISSUES WITH GLOBAL REPORTING OF SUICIDE

Official figures for suicide may not be comparable between WHO member states, nor between regions within those states. Counts of suicides are based on death certificates signed by legally authorized professionals, usually doctors or police officers, or, in the UK, coroner's conclusions. Suicides are often underreported (by 20 to 100 per cent) for social or religious reasons (Bertolote and Fleishmann, 2002). Additionally, different countries have different definitions of suicide or different burdens of proof.

NOMENCLATURE

The above sections have used a number of terms that now need to be defined and explored further.

IS THE TERM 'NON-COMMUNICABLE' THE SAME AS 'CHRONIC' OR 'LONG-TERM'?

No, though the terms are frequently used interchangeably. Non-communicable diseases are those where there is no person-to-person ('horizontal') transmission, by means, for example, of micro-organisms. The presence of microorganisms has been implicated in the causation of some non-communicable diseases (such as *Helicobacter pylori* in stomach cancer), but it is not currently thought that such conditions are transmissible from person to person. Genetic susceptibility to many of these conditions is, however, vertically transmissible – from parent to offspring (see section on the 'thrifty genotype' hypothesis below).

Note that the medical use of the term 'chronic' refers to time rather than severity. A 'chronic condition' is one that lasts 'some time' (variously defined). Its opposite is 'acute', which, again, in medical parlance means 'sudden' rather than 'severe'. 'Chronic' and 'long-term' are, thus, synonymous. Note also that some communicable diseases (such as HIV/AIDS and TB) can be long-term and some non-communicable diseases (such as ischaemic heart disease) can have apparently acute onsets.

WHAT IS THE DEFINITION OF 'INJURIES'?

The definition 'physical damage to a person caused by an acute transfer of energy … or by sudden absence of heat or oxygen' has been broadened to include damage that results in 'psychological harm, maldevelopment, or deprivation' (Norton and Kobusingye, 2013).

Injuries are frequently divided into 'unintentional' (mainly the results of road traffic injuries, falls, drowning or fires) and 'intentional' (self-harm, interpersonal violence and war and other conflict).

WHAT ARE SUICIDAL BEHAVIOURS?

Suicidal behaviours range from suicidal ideation to planning suicide, attempting suicide, completing suicide and intentionally taking one's own life. They are a cause of distress for many people – the individual, family, friends, professionals and the community at large. Up to 19 people in every 100 will have thoughts of suicide at some point in their lives (Weissman et al., 1999), but few of those who harm themselves or think about suicide will actually die through suicide.

Although suicide is quite rare, every year almost 800,000 people die as a result of suicide around the world: 2 per cent of deaths worldwide (WHO, 2014). While suicide is a serious problem in HICs, LMICs bear the larger part of the global suicide burden. Men are approximately three times more likely to take their own lives than women. The most commonly used methods for suicide are firearms, poisons, knives, drowning, hanging, suffocation and jumping from heights. Ingestion of pesticides is commonly used in LIC. Women are more likely to engage in non-fatal suicidal behaviours that require hospital admission.

WHAT IS THE DEFINITION OF 'SELF-HARM'?

It is usually defined as intentional self-poisoning or self-injury, irrespective of the nature of the motivation for doing it or degree of suicidal intent. The method, nature of the motivation or degree of suicidal intent is complex and may change for any individual over time. Long-term outcome studies in adults consistently highlight the association between self-harm and suicide (Suominen et al., 2004). Those who repeat self-harm are at significantly greater risk of suicide than those who have a single episode.

It can be difficult to differentiate behaviours where there is an intent to die (cutting with suicidal intent) from those where there is a pattern of self-harm with no suicidal intent (habitual self-cutting). Also, the method, motivation and intent may change for any individual over time.

Self-harm is an important public health problem in its own right, regardless of intent. It is one of the top five causes of hospital admissions in HICs and one of the top 20 for DALYs.

Activity 10.3

Read the following case histories and note the main learning points. Both of these case histories are based on real cases, to which some further details have been added in order to draw out a larger number of learning points.

Case history 1

Coronary heart disease, type 2 diabetes, traditional healers, economic pressure and self-harm.

Mr R. lived in Bangalore, India. He was married with four children. The eldest daughter and the son had married and left home, though they still lived in Bangalore. The two youngest daughters lived at home with Mr R. and his wife. Mr R. was a street fruit seller.

At the age of 41, Mr R. was admitted to a public hospital in Bangalore with a 'mild heart attack'. While he was in hospital, he was diagnosed as having type 2 diabetes. He was discharged and told he needed 500 mg of metformin twice per day to control his diabetes. He went to see a GP once and, from then on, purchased this metformin from his local pharmacy.

As time went on (he was now 46 years old), he developed a leg ulcer. He visited a local traditional healer, who advised him to stop the metformin and apply a honey-based paste to the ulcer. Despite this, the ulcer failed to heal and, over a matter of weeks, became infected and began to be evil-smelling. As a result of this, no one would buy fruit at his stall and the family income fell drastically. Despairing of the traditional healer, he went to see a second GP who advised him (wrongly) that the only treatment for him was amputation of his leg below the knee and told him (also wrongly) this treatment would cost him the equivalent of half his annual wage from his fruit trade.

After a week or so of worry, declining health and declining income, Mr R. decided that the only course of action was for him to go down to the railway tracks behind their house

(Continued)

(Continued)

and lay his leg across the rails so that a train could amputate his leg. This he did, late one night. The resultant trauma to his leg, hip and pelvis and the consequent blood loss were fatal. He was found in the morning at the side of the track.

Case history 2

Suicide, underreporting, alcohol use, impulsivity, depression, social isolation, substance misuse, single vehicle/ single occupancy collision.

P., who was 17 at the time of his death, lived in a small town in Wales, UK. He was the eldest of four children of Mr S., a nurse, and his wife, a part-time teaching assistant.

P.'s last year in education had not been a happy one and his attendance had become increasingly poor. P. left school at 16 with few qualifications and was considering starting a plumbing course. Most of P.'s friends had stayed on in school, including his girlfriend of the last six months. There was minor conflict between P. and his parents regarding his lack of direction and P. was being encouraged to find some work to give his day some structure.

When P. was 12, his father's brother had taken his own life after being made redundant and separating from his wife.

In the week prior to his death, P. and his girlfriend had split up following an encounter with another girl at a party where P. had been drinking and smoking cannabis. P. had been begging his girlfriend to take him back and had sent text messages saying he 'could not go on without her'. None of his friends considered these to be serious threats. P. had been seeing less and less of his old school friends in the couple of months prior to his death.

On the night of his death, P. had been at home all day, then gone to the house of a friend whom he had met since leaving school and where he had drunk alcohol. On returning home in the early evening, he argued with his father about starting his course. P. left the house in the middle of this and, unknown to his parents, took the family car. P. had been having driving lessons with his father. At some point after this, P. texted his ex-girlfriend, telling her he loved her and not to blame herself.

P. was found dead later that evening in the family car following a collision with a tree on a quiet country road not far from where he lived. He had not been wearing his seat belt. The coroner's conclusion was that of an accidental death.

Comment

You may have taken different learning points from these two cases.

Case history 1

- Early onset of cardiovascular disease in people of South Asian origin.
- Diagnosis of type 2 diabetes while being treated for myocardial infarction is common. Hyperglycaemia might be, in part, the result of this, but also might be indicative of long-standing, undiagnosed hyperglycaemia.
- Type 2 diabetes is becoming commoner in many developing countries and affecting economically active sectors of the community.

- Health systems in many countries are orientated towards acute conditions, but not long-term conditions, such as the non-communicable diseases of cardiovascular disease, respiratory disease, cancer and diabetes. Mr R. did not have a usual GP, he shopped around.
- Universal health coverage is not available in many countries, hence the cost of treatment falls on third-party payers, such as health insurance companies or, as in the case of the underinsured or uninsured, on the individual and the family. This financial stress, on top of physical illness, can lead to tragic consequences. Ironically, Mr R. could have received treatment for his ulcer or, if required, amputation, at a public hospital.
- Traditional healers are often consulted in LMICs, their advice often being taken in addition to that of 'Western'-style medical authorities. They pose a particular risk to patients when effective 'Western'-style therapies are abandoned in favour of traditional therapies of questionable effectiveness and variable dosage.
- This is an example of 'self-harm', albeit misguided 'self-therapy'.

Case history 2

- After accidents, suicide is the second leading cause of death in the 15 to 19 years age group.
- Evidence-based risk factors for suicide in adolescents are male gender, restricted educational achievement, interpersonal difficulties, including connectedness with peers, depression and drug and alcohol misuse.
- Gatekeeper and peer training in suicide awareness may enable people to both recognize and respond appropriately to those who express suicidal thoughts.
- A family history of suicidal behaviour increases the risk of suicide. Providing support to family and close friends following a bereavement through suicide is an important aspect of individual management and prevention (called post-vention).
- Some probable suicides are recorded in official statistics as accidents or misadventure. Where intent is not determined, many official statistics will count the death as a probable suicide, but, in adults, accidental hangings, poisonings (excluding those with narcotics) and single occupancy, single vehicle collisions may be counted as possible suicides.

COMMON FACTORS IN THE GLOBAL EPIDEMIC OF NON-COMMUNICABLE DISEASES, INJURIES, SUICIDE AND SELF-HARM

The extent of the current global epidemic is determined by the following.

- **An ageing population** The proportion of people aged 65 years plus is increasing, so both the incidence and prevalence of cardiovascular disease, chronic lung disease, the major cancers and type 2 diabetes rise as a consequence.
- **Urbanization** The proportion of people living in urban rather than rural environments is increasing, particularly in LMICs. This increasing urbanization has resulted in:
  o decreased physical activity, leading to being overweight and obesity
  o qualitative dietary changes, particularly related to an increased intake of fat (particularly saturated fat and trans-fats), sugar and salt
  o decrease in dietary fibre (non-starch polysaccharide) consumption

o an increase in tobacco and alcohol consumption

o increased risk of transportation-related injuries

o increased exposure to potentially harmful occupational situations and sub-stances

o 'status incongruity' and other related psychosocial stresses, such as social isolation resulting from the break-up of extended families, competition for employment, living space and the threat of crime and violence.

- **Improved healthcare** In many communities, despite health services being largely focused on acute care rather than prevention and long-term care, tangible improve-ments in access to care, increased and earlier diagnosis of non-communicable diseases and better therapy and rehabilitation in some environments and for some groups within society exist.

QUANTIFYING THE EFFECTS OF INDIVIDUAL RISK FACTORS

The contributions of some of these environmental risk factors to non-communicable disease DALYs worldwide have been estimated by Beaglehole and Yach (2003), as shown in Table 10.4.

A history of self-harm and the presence of a mental health disorder are the pre-dominant risk factors for suicidal behaviours. Approximately 90 per cent of those

Table 10.4 Contributions of various environmental risk factors to DALYs worldwide

		Developing countries			
Developed countries		High mortality**		Low mortality**	
Risk factor	% of total DALYs	Risk factor	% of total DALYs	Risk factor	% of total DALYs
Tobacco	12.14	Underweight	14.0	Alcohol	6.3
Blood pressure	11.0	Unsafe sex	11.7	Underweight	5.8
Alcohol	9.3	Unsafe water etc.	5.6	Blood pressure	5.0
Cholesterol*	7.6	Indoor smoke	3.8	Tobacco	4.2
Body mass index	7.5	Zinc deficiency	3.3	Body mass index	2.7
Low fruit and vegetable intake	3.9	Iron deficiency	3.2	Cholesterol*	2.1
Physical inactivity	3.3	Vitamin A deficiency	2.9	Iron deficiency	2.0
Illicit drugs	1.9	Blood pressure	2.5	Low fruit and vegetable intake	1.9
Underweight	1.3	Tobacco	1.9	Indoor smoke	1.9
Iron deficiency	0.8	Cholesterol*	1.9	Unsafe water, etc.	1.8

*Refers to serum cholesterol, particularly low-density lipoprotein cholesterol (LDL).

**Low-mortality developing countries include, for example, China, Brazil and Thailand. High-mortality developing countries include India, Mali and Nigeria.

Source: Beaglehole and Yach (2003)

who die through suicide have a psychiatric diagnosis at the time of death (Bertolote and Fleishman, 2002). Other factors consistently associated with suicide include physical illness, alcohol and substance misuse, acute emotional stress and major changes in individuals' lives, such as separation and divorce or loss of employment. Usually it is a complex combination of these factors (health, social, economic and cultural issues) that contributes to this tragic event (Table 10.5).

Table 10.5   Risk factors associated with suicide

Factor	Estimated increased risk to general population where known
Male	x 3
Current or ex-psychiatric patient	x 10
4 weeks following discharge from a psychiatric hospital	x 100–200
Prisoners	x 5–10
Self-harm	x 30
In first year following self-harm	x 66
>60 years with more than one episode of self-harm requiring hospital treatment	x 49
>60 years with a bereavement in the last year	x 3.5
Drug misuse	x 20
Alcohol misuse	x 6
Physical illness (cancer, multiple sclerosis, epilepsy, chronic pain)	Not known
Unemployment	x 2–3
Male divorce or separation	x 2
Family history of suicide	Not known

Source: National Health Wales (2008)

'NATURE' AND 'NURTURE' EFFECTS ON NON-COMMUNICABLE DISEASES

THE 'THRIFTY GENOTYPE' HYPOTHESIS

Many non-communicable diseases have increased suddenly and markedly over the past 75 years or so, in particular the cardiovascular diseases ischaemic heart disease, stroke and hypertension, plus type 2 diabetes and obesity. These increases have occurred in association with the rapid social transformations of urbanization and Westernization.

In 1962, geneticist J.V. Neel proposed the 'thrifty genotype' hypothesis, whereby, in conditions of hunter-gathering and 'feast and famine' subsistence economies, a significant selective advantage favoured individuals who carried the genetic potential for obesity, type 2 diabetes and, indirectly, cardiovascular diseases. In former times, the phenotypic disadvantages of these diseases did not become manifest because of the relatively low energy density of the diet, the high levels of physical activity needed to survive and low life expectancy. With rapid transformation of the environment and the consequent intake of high-energy foods, lower levels of energy expenditure and longer life expectancy, this genetic predisposition led to high frequencies of the conditions and phenotypic disadvantage.

THE 'THRIFTY PHENOTYPE' HYPOTHESIS

Some retrospective cohort studies have reported an association between low birthweight (corrected for gestational age) and a high risk of the occurrence of hypertension and type 2 diabetes (and related impaired glucose tolerance) and mortality from cardiovascular disease in adult life. This association is compounded by the development in adult life of being overweight and obesity so that the individuals at highest risk are those who are born small and later become overweight or obese.

That low birthweight of offspring is a consequence of poor nutrition of the mother during pregnancy has long been known in animal husbandry and animal experiments. This effect is transgenerational – that is, low birthweight female offspring of nutritionally compromised animals tend to have offspring with relatively low birthweights, even when the nutritional environment of their pregnancies is adequate.

The study of some famines resulting from natural disasters and wars (the Dutch winter famine of 1944 to 1945, for example), has shown a similar transgenerational effect that gradually diminishes over time. It is not entirely clear which trimester of pregnancy is the most critical for this effect to be generated.

Activity 10.4

Find recent articles on the above two hypotheses and assess the credibility of either, neither or both as explanations or partial explanations for the pattern of non-communicable diseases we see worldwide today.

WORLDWIDE STRATEGIES FOR PREVENTION

The most formidable public health challenge is the prevention of LTCs. Potentially all can be prevented or at least delayed in their onset. The optimistic view would point out that many preventive strategies are common to more than one condition. The pessimistic view would have it that none of the potential preventive measures is straightforward – there's no certain way of decreasing tobacco use. Ample evidence from some countries, however, is that it is possible to do so, given the convergence of a number of strategies, each of which would be virtually ineffective without the others.

Preventive strategies in relation to psychiatric disorders occur at three levels:

- *universal* approaches, targeting the whole population
- *selective* approaches, targeting subgroups that possess one or more risk factors
- *indicated* approaches, targeting specific individuals who are at risk (Mrazek and Haggerty, 1994).

These terms can be applied to many of the conditions addressed in this chapter.

TOBACCO CONTROL – THE WHO'S TOBACCO FREE INITIATIVE

The most important measures in the prevention of lung cancer and chronic lung disease are those directed towards decreased use of tobacco and decreased exposure to tobacco smoke, among both smokers and non-smokers ('passive smoking'). Such measures are also very likely to contribute to the prevention of ischaemic heart disease, hypertension and stroke. Also, eliminating smoking during pregnancy reduces the risk of growth retardation of the foetus, leading to the birth of babies who are small for their gestational age. Some evidence exists that smoking during pregnancy increases the risk of the later development of type 2 diabetes in the offspring (possibly related to the 'thrifty phenotype hypothesis'). Thus, a reduction in smoking during pregnancy may also contribute to a reduction in the incidence of type 2 diabetes.

In terms of the three categories of prevention, universal approaches, directed at the entire population, include measures to reduce or eliminate the advertising of tobacco products and legislation relating to pricing. Selective approaches include those directed at specific populations, such as young people at risk of taking up smoking and pregnant women in whom smoking would pose risks to not only themselves but also the unborn foetus. Indicated approaches include pharmaceutical and other management initiatives to enable existing smokers to quit.

National approaches to tobacco control generally aim to:

- eliminate tobacco advertising, whether totally, in connection with sporting or other public events, at particularly sensitive sites (such as near schools) or everywhere except at the point of sale
- eliminate or severely restrict sponsorship of events (such as sporting events) by tobacco product manufacturers
- use fiscal pricing mechanisms of tobacco products as disincentives to continuing or starting smoking
- label tobacco products with messages about the health dangers of smoking
- legislate against smoking in enclosed public spaces
- direct public information campaigns targeted towards specific social groups, such as young people or pregnant women
- encourage health professionals to provide support to existing smokers who wish to quit
- provide information on over-the-counter measures to assist those who wish to quit

These and other measures are summarized in the WHO *Framework Convention on Tobacco Control* (2003).

DIET AND PHYSICAL ACTIVITY – CONTROLLING THE GLOBAL OBESITY EPIDEMIC

Urbanization has contributed to the emergence of several non-communicable diseases through being overweight and obese. Excess bodyweight (particularly abdominal obesity) directly relates to risk of type 2 diabetes and contributes to elevated risk of ischaemic heart disease, hypertension (and, thereby, stroke), as well as other debilitating conditions, such as osteoarthritis. There is also accumulating evidence linking being overweight and obese to breast and colon cancers.

Universal approaches encourage the general population to increase levels of physical activity and avoid foods high in fat and refined carbohydrates.

Selective approaches are directed towards those at particularly high risk, such as children and women during pregnancy. Many countries face the challenge of the two extremes of under- and over-nutrition simultaneously in different sectors of the community. Indicated approaches aim to reduce the weight of those already within the overweight or obese categories by therapeutic means – lifestyle interventions, pharmacological interventions or, in extreme cases, bariatric surgery.

National approaches to controlling the obesity epidemic include:

- encouraging people to make healthy choices through public awareness campaigns
- enabling individuals to make these healthy choices, such as improved food labelling
- legislation to control the amounts of saturated fat, trans fats, salt and refined carbohydrates (such as sucrose) in foods and drinks
- initiatives focused on children, pregnant women and other vulnerable groups to encourage healthy eating and physical activity in schools and other settings.

These and other measures are summarized in the WHO's (n.d.) *Global Strategy on Diet, Physical Activity and Health*.

ROAD TRAFFIC INJURY PREVENTION

As one of the most important causes of injury, in both the developed and developing world, road traffic incidents ('accidents' is regarded as a misleading term) have been the focus of a number of global, regional and national prevention initiatives. Universal approaches aimed at reducing the frequency and severity of these incidents include population-wide campaigns to improve road safety among drivers and pedestrians, while selective approaches target drivers specifically to encourage drink-, drug- and fatigue-free driving and the observance of speed limits and other driving laws. Indicated approaches include measures to rehabilitate drivers who have transgressed these laws by means of specific driving awareness courses in lieu of or in addition to fines or imprisonment.

National approaches to reducing the frequency and severity of traffic injuries include:

- better land use and transport planning – by providing shorter and safer pedestrian and cycle routes, together with convenient, safe and affordable public transport
- improved road design, incorporating, where appropriate, traffic calming measures, controlled crossings for pedestrians and adequate street lighting
- legislation to enforce the wearing of seat belts, cycle helmets and child restraints
- the adequate enforcement of speed limits, other driving regulations and curbs on driving under the influence of alcohol, drugs or when fatigued.

These and other measures are summarized in the WHO's (2004) *World Report on Road Traffic Injury Prevention*.

SUICIDE AND SELF-HARM PREVENTION – BEYOND HEALTH SERVICES

Suicide prevention is a global public health challenge. Common universal suicide prevention programmes include gatekeeper training programmes for those coming into contact with vulnerable people, peer support programmes, skills development programmes and suicide awareness education programmes. Selective suicide prevention programmes usually involve risk screening to identify those with one or more risk factors, such as depression and unemployment followed by early intervention or treatment programmes.

A common indicated suicide prevention approach is to help those at risk, such as those who have self-harmed or who have suicidal ideation. Suicide prevention requires a cross-governmental department approach that is broader than mental health services – including health and social care, economics, housing, transport, justice and substance misuse – combined with an awareness of particular settings, such as schools, prisons, hospitals, railways, or bridges.

National approaches to suicide prevention generally aim to:

- promote early identification, assessment, treatment and appropriate referral to professional care of people at risk of suicidal behaviour (including those with mental health disorders and self-harm behaviours)
- increase public and professional access to information on preventing suicidal behaviour
- establish integrated data collection to identify at risk groups, individuals and situations
- promote public awareness and understanding of mental well-being and suicidal behaviour to encourage people to seek help and ensure there is appropriate community-level support
- maintain a comprehensive training programme for identified gatekeepers (such as police, educators, social workers, mental health professionals)
- promote appropriate public reporting and portrayal of suicide and suicidal behaviour
- provide support and effective services for people affected by suicide and suicidal behaviours
- reduce the availability, accessibility and attractiveness of the means to suicidal behaviour
- establish institutions or agencies to promote or coordinate research, training and service delivery with respect to suicidal behaviours.

The WHO has set out a public health approach to suicide prevention (WHO, 2014).

Lack of mental well-being underpins many physical diseases, unhealthy lifestyles and social inequalities in health. Mental health and physical health should be treated with 'parity of esteem' to reduce the effects of these major health problems.

CONCLUSION

This chapter has explained the terms 'non-communicable diseases', 'injuries', 'suicide' and 'self-harm' and discussed the considerable extent to which these conditions contribute to the global burden of disease.

The measures by which these contributions have been measured are DALYs, YLLs and YLDs and these provide instruments for comparing the impact of non-communicable disease and long-term conditions on health services and systems.

The contributions of major environmental risk factors to this burden have also been explored and quantified and it has been noted that several of these risk factors are related to more than one condition, as tobacco use is to chronic lung diseases, lung cancer and ischaemic heart disease.

A public health, preventive approach is needed worldwide to help eliminate or reduce the risk factors. Mental health and well-being are closely related to the extent to which individuals are able to respond to these preventive measures. Public health strategies and other global initiatives relevant to the management and prevention of these conditions are advocated by the WHO and other similar organizations, with the basic tenet being to 'think globally and act locally'.

REFERENCES

Beaglehole, R. and Yach, D. (2003) 'Globalisation and the prevention and control of non-communicable disease: the neglected chronic diseases of adults', *The Lancet*, 362: 903–908.

Bertolote, J.M. and Fleishman, A. (2002) 'Suicide and psychiatric diagnosis: a worldwide perspective', *World Psychiatry*, 1(3): 181–185.

Buonaguro, F.M., Gueye, S.N., Wabinga, H.R., Ngoma, T.A., Vermorken, J.B. and Mbulaitaye, S.M. (2013) 'Clinical oncology in resource-limited settings', *Infectious Agents and Cancer*, 8: 39.

Mrazek, P.J. and Haggerty, R.J. (eds) (1994) *Committee on Prevention of Mental Disorders; Institute of Medicine. Reducing Risks for Mental Disorders: Frontiers for Preventive Intervention Research*. The National Academies Press.

Murray, C.J., Vos, T., Lozano, R. et al. (2012) 'Disability-adjusted life years (DALYs) for 291 diseases and injuries in 21 regions, 1990–2010: a systematic analysis for the Global Burden of Disease Study 2010', *The Lancet*; 380: 2197–2223.

National Health Service Wales (2008) *NPHS Briefing on Suicide in Wales*, 7 February. Available at: www.wales.nhs.uk/sitesplus/888/news/14542 (accessed 1 October 2015).

Norton, R. and Kobusingye, O. (2013) 'Injuries', *N Engl J Med*, 368: 1723–1729.

Nugent, R.A. and Feigl, A.B. (2010) *Where Have All the Donors Gone? Scarce Donor Funding for Non-Communicable Diseases*. Working Paper No. 228. Available at: http://dspace.cigilibrary.org/jspui/handle/123456789/30109 (accessed 8 October 2015).

Suominen, K.D., Isometsä, E., Suokas, J. et al. (2004) 'Completed suicide after a suicide attempt: a 37-year follow-up study', *Am J Psychiatry*, 161: 562–563.

Weissman, M.M., Bland, R.C., Canino, G.J. et al. (1999) 'Prevalence of suicide ideation and suicide attempts in nine countries', *Psychological Medicine*, 29: 9–17.

World Health Organization (n.d.) *Global Strategy on Diet, Physical Activity and Health*. Available at: www.who.int/dietphysicalactivity/en (accessed 1 October 2015).

World Health Organization (2003) *WHO Framework Convention on Tobacco Control*. Geneva: WHO. Available at: www.who.int/fctc/text_download/en/ (accessed 30 June 2015).

World Health Organization (2004) *World Report on Road Traffic Injury Prevention*. Geneva: WHO. Available at: www.who.int/violence_injury_prevention/publications/road_traffic/world_report/en/ (accessed 30 June 2015).

World Health Organization (2005) *Preventing Chronic Diseases: A Vital Investment*. Geneva: WHO.

World Health Organization (2014) *Preventing Suicide: A Global Imperative*. Geneva: WHO. Available at: http://apps.who.int/iris/bitstream/10665/131056/1/9789241564779_eng.pdf?ua=1 (accessed 8 October 2015).

11

MENTAL HEALTH, MENTAL ILLNESS AND DISABILITY

SUBODH DAVE, RACHEL JENKINS AND NISHA DOGRA

Chapter overview

After reading this chapter, you should be able to:

- describe the global importance of mental health and mental illness within differing sociocultural contexts
- describe the impact of mental illness on physical morbidity, disability and mortality
- examine global disparities in resources for the care of people with mental illness
- identify ways of addressing mental health and mental illness in different resource environments.

INTRODUCTION

This chapter defines mental health and mental illness in different cultural contexts. The impact of stigma on how individuals with mental illness are viewed and the services available to them are described. It demonstrates that mental illness and its impact is a serious global concern that requires urgent intervention. The chapter concludes with suggestions for steps that can be taken to improve the outcomes of care for mentally ill people.

─────────────────── Activity 11.1 ───────────────────

What words or images do you associate with the following terms:

- mental health
- mental health problems

(Continued)

(Continued)

- mental illness
- mental disorder.

How would you be able to tell if someone was experiencing mental health problems or mental illness?

Comment

You may have found it difficult to differentiate between these terms because they seem to overlap. The following section unpacks these concepts.

CONCEPTS OF MENTAL HEALTH, ILLNESS AND DISORDER

There is a range of confusing terminology around mental health and mental illness. Often terms are used to avoid stigmatization (discussed below) but the effect is that prejudice is pandered to and confusion arises.

DEFINING MENTAL HEALTH

Mental health is a term that may be used, both in the literature and in verbal communication, to refer to positive mental health (such as happiness, well-being, resilience) or to mental disorders (such as depression, anxiety or schizophrenia) or to a continuum of experience from positive mental health to mental disorder. It is therefore important in communications to work out in what sense the term is being used. The WHO (2007) states that:

> Mental Health refers to a broad array of activities directly or indirectly related to the mental well-being component included in the WHO's definition of health: 'A state of complete physical, mental and social well-being, and not merely the absence of disease'. It is related to the promotion of well-being, the prevention of mental disorders, and the treatment and rehabilitation of people affected by mental disorders.

Mental health is a status in itself, not just the result of the absence of illness. An individual with 'good' mental health can function effectively in social relationships and in the workplace. Despite this, the WHO observes that even less funding is available for mental health promotion (as compared to funding for service provision for mental illness) aimed at having a positive effect on well-being in general. The encouragement of individual resources and skills and improvements in the socio-economic environment are among the strategies used to promote good mental health. Mental health promotion requires multi-sectoral action involving several stakeholders. The focus should be on promoting mental health throughout the individual's lifespan in order to ensure a healthy start in life for children and prevent mental disorders in adulthood and old age (WHO, 2007).

MENTAL HEALTH PROBLEMS

This term has gained widespread use to avoid stigmatizing those who have some problems with their mental health. It is sometimes used to indicate 'problems' that are less severe and below the threshold of the diagnostic criteria using one of the two major classification systems, namely the *International Classification of Diseases* (ICD) or *Diagnostic and Statistical Manual of Mental Disorders* (DSM).

The term 'mental health problem' covers a wide range of problems that affect someone's ability to get on with their daily life. Mental health problems and, indeed, frank mental disorder can affect anyone, of any age and background, as well as having an impact on the people around them, such as their family, friends and carers. Mental health problems and mental disorders result from a complex interaction of biological, social and psychological factors. Major life events, such as bereavement, relationship break-up or serious illness, can impact significantly how we feel about ourselves and, subsequently, our mental state and health. Thus, in addition to biological factors, psychosocial factors play a significant role in the onset and severity of mental health problems and mental illness, and in their maintenance and recovery.

MENTAL DISORDER AND MENTAL ILLNESS

A mental illness is an illness comprising disturbances in thinking, perception and behaviour, which are not developmentally or socially normative. The disturbances can be mild, moderate or severe and may seriously interfere with a person's life, significantly impairing a person's ability to cope with life's ordinary demands and routines. They are often associated with disability and increased risk of mortality.

Mental disorder is common, occurring in approximately 10 per cent of children and 15 per cent of adults at any one time. 'Mental disorder' is a broad term, legally defined as, 'any disorder or disability of the mind' in the Mental Health Act (2007) of England and Wales. Clinically, it is often used in the sense that a person who is mentally ill is suffering from a mental disorder that fulfils the diagnostic criteria set out in the ICD and DSM diagnostic frameworks.

Diagnostic concepts are further complicated as there can be differences between what is objectively observed and what is subjectively perceived or experienced. For example, using the criteria required to meet the diagnostic frameworks, a clinician may diagnose a mild or moderate anxiety disorder, but, for the patient, the impact on his or her life may be significant. Equally, seriously mentally ill people – those suffering from mania or acute psychoses, for example – may display overtly abnormal behaviour, but may subjectively believe themselves to be well.

This has led some to challenge the very construct 'mental disorder'. The challenges include the rejection of mental illness for lacking a physical pathology, individualizing and pathologizing social distress and ignoring the political dimension of mental illness (Thomas and Bracken, 2004). It has been argued that 'mental health' might usefully be viewed as a continuum of experience, from mental well-being through to a severe and enduring mental illness. There is increasing research evidence, however, that well-being and mental illness are not on a single continuum, but form two different dimensions of experience (Manderscheid et al., 2010).

Psychosocial factors and their influence on the development or maintenance of mental health problems and mental disorders vary according to context. The quality of a person's mental health is influenced by idiosyncratic individual factors and experiences, family relationships, the wider community and the cultural environment in which he or she lives. People's cultural backgrounds can affect:

- the way they think about mental health and mental health problems and make sense of certain symptoms and behaviours
- the way their families and communities respond to them when they're ill
- their illness behaviour, such as sickness absence, over-the-counter medication, prescribed medication
- the services they choose to seek, such as traditional medicine, primary care or specialist care
- the treatment and management strategies they find acceptable
- the way in which those who have mental health problems are perceived by the family, community, health workers and service planners.

Epilepsy, for example, is considered a mental illness in some parts of the world. Such classifications may change when more medical explanations are adopted, but using Western norms to classify mental disorders risks the loss of the rich sociocultural context relevant to the understanding of such disorders.

STIGMA

The stigmatization of mental illness is a worldwide phenomenon (Crisp, 2004) and individuals with mental illness continue to face a wide range of problems because of the negative attitudes towards them.

Stigmatization is a social construct whereby those with mental illness are identified as being different and having less worth. 'Stigma' can be defined as the co-occurrence of its components and effects: labelling, stereotyping, separation, status loss and discrimination. The stigma faced by those with mental illness means that they are often ostracized from society and fail to receive the care they require. Even when they receive care, it may be associated with deprivation of basic human rights, abuse and neglect, as evidenced by the sight of patients restrained with metal shackles or confined in caged beds (WHO, 2006).

Discrimination may be systematized in law. In some countries, those with mental illness are prohibited from voting, marrying or having children. Discrimination in the form of lack of opportunities for education and employment is almost universal.

The many campaigns to change negative attitudes and raise awareness – Every Family in the Land, for example – have had limited effect (Crisp, 2004). The lack of success may relate to inadequate funding and negative attitudes, not just of lay people but also of professionals.

─────────────────── Activity 11.2 ───────────────────

List some words that reflect negative attitudes towards patients with mental health problems.
   How do you think you have formed your views on mental illness? If you can, discuss your responses with colleagues.

THE IMPACT OF MENTAL ILLNESS ON THE INDIVIDUAL, THE FAMILY AND THE COMMUNITY

GLOBAL BURDEN OF DISEASE ESTIMATES

Neuropsychiatric disorders form 13 per cent of the Global Burden of Disease and could rise to 15 per cent by 2020. They comprise five of the ten leading causes of disability, and account for 28 per cent of years of life lived with a disability (YLDs). Depression alone is expected to rise from being the fourth to the second leading cause of the global disease burden by 2030. It will be the leading cause of disability in HICs, second only to HIV/AIDS in MICs and third only to HIV/AIDS and perinatal conditions in LICs. Suicide (the majority of cases being linked with depression) was the tenth leading cause of death (see Chapter 10). These figures do not take account of the burden on families or the wider social and economic impacts.

PREVALENCE OF MENTAL DISORDERS

Annual global prevalence rates are estimated at around 5 to 15 per cent for common mental disorders and 2 per cent for psychosis. Half of common mental disorders last for longer than one year, unless they are adequately treated. Two thirds of people with psychosis experience a relapsing or deteriorating course, unless adequately treated. Substance and alcohol abuse rates and learning difficulties are also common across the globe. Progressive organic diseases of the brain (dementia) have been found to affect around 5 per cent of people aged 65 plus in some Asian and Latin American countries. Dementia is expected to become increasingly common in LMICs as overall life expectancy increases and because as much as 90 per cent of the burden of HIV/AIDS is in LMICs, with the attendant problem of HIV-related dementia.

ASSOCIATION WITH PHYSICAL ILLNESS AND MORTALITY

Mental disorders are associated with increased mortality and physical morbidity. Overall, approximately 60 per cent of excess mortality among people with mental disorders is due to physical health problems, with the most common cause of excess mortality at all ages being cardiovascular disease. The increased risk of mortality from depression alone is similar to that from smoking. Cardiovascular disease is three times more likely and diabetes twice as likely in people with schizophrenia compared to the general population – a problem exacerbated by use of the newer antipsychotic medications, which can cause diabetes, weight gain and metabolic syndrome. Much of this data is from HICs; less is known about the links between poor physical health and mental health in LMICs.

SUICIDE

Suicide is a major cause of death globally. Many poor countries do not have good routine registration of deaths and causes of deaths and few post mortem facilities.

As in some HICs, suicide data may often be collected by the police rather than by health authorities, which may aggravate inconsistencies in reporting. Significant underreporting may also occur, due to the taboo, stigma, religious views and illegality of suicide in some countries.

Premature death from suicide has many adverse consequences. In addition to the loss of life, there is the consequence for the person's family of the loss of a bread-winner or parent, the long-standing psychological trauma for children, friends and relatives, plus the loss of economic productivity for the nation.

In the USA, it is estimated that up to 90 per cent of completed suicides are associated with a mental disorder – a pattern that is likely to be similar globally. Psychological autopsy studies have demonstrated that the so-called rational suicide is extremely rare, with mental illness almost inevitably playing a role.

Non-fatal suicide attempts are associated with significant long-term adverse impacts, as the injuries sustained may lead to disability, a need for family care, loss of income and an elevated risk of future suicidal attempts.

ECONOMIC BURDEN

Mental disorders impose a significant economic burden, not just on the individuals with the disorders but also on their households, communities, employers, primary and secondary healthcare systems and on government budgets. Mental disorders perpetuate the cycle of poverty by interfering with the individual's capacity to func-tion in either paid or non-income roles, leading to decreased social as well as economic productivity. In many LMICs, where universal access to healthcare and financial and social protection systems are often lacking, individuals with mental ill-ness may spend much of their savings or borrow money to manage physical illnesses made more likely by their poverty. Breaking the chain of poverty and debt around mentally ill people is vital to addressing the first of the MDGs – eradicating extreme poverty and hunger.

IMPACT ON THE NEXT GENERATION

Mental disorders affect all ages – about 10 per cent of children and 10 to 15 per cent of young adults experience mental health problems. Longitudinal studies in a number of HICs demonstrate that, untreated, mental health and behavioural problems in childhood and youth can have profound longstanding social and economic consequences in adulthood. These include poorer levels of educa-tional attainment, increased contact with the criminal justice system, reduced levels of employment, lower salaries when employed and personal relationship difficulties.

Mental disorder in parents can adversely impact the health, development and education of their children and the consequences of this influence the presentation of children to PHC. In some LICs, children may be removed from school during health crises to provide informal care for their parent or parents or it may be that the parent or parents are simply too sick to ensure that the children attend school. There are also costs to educational systems for children with unrecognized and untreated mental disorders.

GLOBAL VARIATIONS IN RESOURCES FOR MENTAL HEALTH

The WHO's Mental Health Atlas was developed in 2005 to collect systematic information about country-specific (or region-specific) mental health systems. However, almost a quarter of the world's countries do not have any system for collecting and reporting mental health information. The Mental Health Atlas reveals significant global variation in mental health resources in a range of domains. Key domains for mental health resources globally, as listed by the WHO in its Assessment Instrument for Mental Health Systems (WHO-AIMS), are:

- Domain 1: Policy and legislative framework
- Domain 2: Mental health services
- Domain 3: Mental health in primary healthcare
- Domain 4: Human resources
- Domain 5: Education and links with other sectors
- Domain 6: Monitoring and research.

The overarching message from these mapping exercises is that the allocation of resources to the mental health sector is significantly poor, especially in LMICs (Saxena et al., 2007).

Activity 11.3

Access the World Mental Health Atlas on the WHO's website (at: www.who.int/mental_health/evidence/atlas/mental_health_atlas_2014/en). Choose one HIC and one LIC or MIC and compare them. (A list of LMICs is available at: http://data.worldbank.org/about/country-and-lending-groups#Low_income)

List the main differences between the profiles of the countries you have chosen and discuss these with your colleagues.

THE MENTAL HEALTH POLICY, LEGISLATION AND INTERSECTORIAL LINKAGES

The provision of mental healthcare that meets the needs of the population and works synergistically with the general health system depends on the presence of a mental health policy. A robust mental health policy can facilitate the integration of mental health into health, education, social welfare and criminal justice systems. Regrettably, mental health policy is absent in a third of all countries (over half in Africa). Only 75 per cent of countries have a legislative framework protecting the basic human and civil rights of mentally ill people. Even worse, in some countries, discrimination against mentally ill patients is codified in law. For example, mentally ill people can be excluded from receiving social benefits or from enrolling in health insurance schemes.

Mental healthcare needs to be comprehensive and delivered as close to home as is compatible with the health and safety of the individual and the public. In HICs, asylums have given way to community-based care. Indeed, the median rate of outpatient facilities for mentally ill people in HICs is 58 times that of LICs (WHO, 2011). LMICs often have a large urban mental hospital, but, in rural areas, there is a great shortage of or no acute inpatient beds and outpatient services and scarce capacity for PHC referrals to specialists and in any case the scarcity of specialist staff (see below) means that other solutions are necessary. Home visits may be carried out by interested specialist staff, PHC staff or attached lay volunteers, but are only sporadically present rather than systematically provided for whole populations.

Activity 11.4

List some potential ways in which the deficiencies so far identified might be addressed and what impediments may exist.

Comment

Voluntary organizations in the community try to bridge the gaps in mental health services, but sustained cooperation between governmental and non-governmental organizations is hampered by the lack of policy frameworks to facilitate intersectoral collaboration. Mental health services are also constrained by a lack of patient and carer engagement in the design and delivery of services. This lack is most pronounced in LMICs where, paradoxically, the need is greatest, given the lack of sufficient provision of services from the state sector. However, the mental health NGO sector is much too patchy to be able to make a comprehensive contribution to mental health services across a country.

MENTAL HEALTH IN PHC

It makes sense to integrate mental health into the PHC system because mental disorders are so common and symptoms are usually interwoven with physical symptoms, social problems and contexts. Also, in all countries, but especially in LAMIC, specialists are relatively scarce compared to the numbers of people with mental disorders and PHC is closer to home than specialist care (Jenkins et al., 2013).

Randomized controlled trials show that PHC workers can deliver mental healthcare. One of the major problems is that basic health systems in LMICs are often weak, poorly staffed, poorly supported and supervised, the medicine supply chain is often erratic and health management information systems (HMIS) are often poor. For example, antidepressant medications are unavailable in PHCs in 25 per cent of LMIC countries.

As well as integration of mental health into PHC, integration of mental health into other public health programmes, such as immunization programmes or management of TB or HIV, has been shown to be an effective strategy. There is growing evidence that not only PHC workers but also lay health workers in the community can carry out some of the tasks traditionally carried out by psychiatrists (Patel, 2009).

HUMAN RESOURCES

Good frontline mental healthcare needs close support and supervision from district services and capacity to refer complex cases for assessment and management at district level. Thus, an adequately staffed and trained specialist workforce is also necessary. Such a specialist workforce is also essential for intersectoral collaboration, service planning, audit, research and training.

Funding starvation and stigma related to mental health have, however, led to a chronic shortage of trained professionals in mental health globally, although the problem is far more acute in LMICs. These countries have a median of 0.05 psychiatrists and 0.16 psychiatric nurses per 100,000 of the population (WHO, 2011). In contrast, HICs, such as the UK, have 14 psychiatrists per 100,000 of the population. Overall, the number of mental healthcare workers per capita in HICs is 200 times that of LMICs. This has real consequences for patient care as the lack of sufficient professionals is the main limiting factor when delivering mental healthcare.

Given the overall shortage of over a million mental healthcare workers in LMICs the training agenda is massive (see next section). A range of other initiatives, however, such as task sharing, improving recruitment, improving retention and managing the risk of emigration to HICs, have also been used to address the human resource shortage in mental health.

Another piece of the jigsaw involves collaborations with traditional or faith-based healers/care providers, who constitute a major juncture in the care pathway of mentally ill people, particularly in LMICs (though not exclusively so, as testified by the number of advertisements for faith-based healers in the back pages of Asian/African publications in the UK) (Gureje et al. 2015).

PROFESSIONAL TRAINING

Training professionals in mental healthcare is a key challenge facing the world. The WHO's Atlas project, looking at training in this area all around the world, showed that almost a third of countries lacked any psychiatric training programmes, but, in Africa, this was true for over half of its countries (WHO, 2005). Even in countries where such training programmes exist, the availability of training across the country is patchy. Training in psychotherapy, mental health policy, research or teaching skills and managerial or leadership training were particularly deficient in LMICs.

Where teaching is available, its impact is hampered by the lack of teaching skills, the use of outdated teaching and assessment methods and a misplaced focus on imparting knowledge as opposed to improving skills and attitudes. Notably, self-directed learning was absent in over 75 per cent of countries. Assessment methods also vary, with poor articulation between assessment methods and key learning objectives.

MONITORING AND RESEARCH

Robust evidence is crucial for defining needs, identifying gaps in service design and delivery, designing and implementing clinically sound and cost-effective interventions and, finally, in monitoring the impact of such changes on patient outcomes. Unfortunately, research-based evidence in the context of global mental health is very heavily skewed towards HICs. Applying evidence from research generated in

HICs to LMICs can lead to culturally inappropriate diagnoses and treatments, thus adversely affecting patient outcomes. Reversing this requires not only an improvement in research capacity in LMICs but also the facilitation of wider publication and dissemination of local research through support for authors and editors in these countries.

In sum, global mental health is hit by a triple whammy. It receives a smaller allocation of healthcare resources, the scant resources allocated are inequitably distributed, with the poorest and neediest people left wanting, and, finally, the lack of a proper evidence base means that the meagre resources are often utilized inefficiently (Saxena et al., 2007).

IMPROVING GLOBAL MENTAL HEALTH

While the focus of the previous section may have been on LMICs, access to good mental healthcare is a global problem. The 'treatment gap' (the proportion of people affected by a mental disorder not receiving any treatment whatsoever), even in the HICs of Europe and in the USA, is estimated to be over 67 per cent. In LMICs, this figure approaches 90 per cent (Lancet Mental Health Group, 2007).

Clearly, scaling up human and financial resources globally for mental health will be a crucial aspect of the solution, but merely enhancing resources is not sufficient, as shown by the fact that there is a treatment gap in HICs. Numerous examples of cost-effective solutions identified in LMICs have global relevance, including for HICs. Turning the World Upside Down (TTWUD) is a recent endeavour that disseminates such projects (see Activity 11.5 below).

Activity 11.5

Go to the TTWUD website (at: www.ttwud.org). Find 'The Dream-A-World Cultural Therapy intervention for promoting resilience in High Risk Primary School Children in Jamaica' (click on the 'Mental health' button on the home page), read it and discuss with friends how you might apply the ideas in your country. Think about the barriers you might face and the steps needed to overcome them.

Comment

Your ideas will be very context-specific, so we cannot imagine what your answer is, but we expect you will be able to apply the following framework of:

- identifying need, context and constraints
- securing support through advocacy and liaising with key stakeholders
- agreeing policy and strategy
- planning outcome-based activities
- securing resources
- implementing and monitoring activities
- evaluating impact
- disseminating findings.

CORE STEPS TO TAKE TO ADDRESS THE BURDEN OF MENTAL DISORDERS

To address mental disorders, it is important that the issue should be recognized by policymakers. As PHC is the level at which persons suffering from mental disorders are likely to present first, it is important that healthcare workers at that level are trained to recognize the signs and know when to refer people to a system that is supported by resources allowing for specialist provision.

POLICY STEPS

The design and implementation of a robust mental health policy requires strong advocacy, encouragement by major donors and support from relevant ministers or local champions, as well as civil servants inside the Ministry of Health who are able to translate such a vision into legislation. Generating such political will on a global basis is not unheard of. At one time, programmes for AIDS/HIV suffered from widespread stigma and apathy, but concerted global action and partnerships across state and non-governmental sectors have transformed the fate of HIV sufferers across the world. Mental health is worthy of similar concerted global action. The sheer number of mentally ill people in the world being denied fundamental and universal human rights, such as freedom and the right to care, requires a global policy response.

INTEGRATION OF MENTAL HEALTH INTO THE PHC SYSTEM

A stepped care model, with treatment of people with mild and moderately severe disorders at PHC level and referral of the most challenging cases to more specialist workers (the relative proportions dependent on availability of services), is an effective way to address capacity issues. It is feasible and practicable to integrate mental health into PHC, accompanied by good practice guidelines, and achieve good outcomes in LICs (Jenkins et al., 2013).

Moreover, effective integration of mental health into other health programmes, such as those for HIV, TB, malaria, child health and reproductive health, and, more widely, with other non-health sectors, such as education, social welfare, the criminal justice system and the NGO sectors, could enhance client focus and improve efficiency of the delivery of care. Yet, in many settings, effective integration is difficult to achieve as it requires political commitment, time for joint planning and appropriate training of staff so that health professionals consider holistic management of patients as part of their roles and responsibilities.

Unfortunately, the lack of leadership and public health expertise and the lack of evaluation and outcome measures at the outset when implementing new mental health programmes (80 per cent of the programmes in Africa had no evaluation statistics) has hampered such integration. Effective supervision and leadership, with inclusion of mental health outcomes in routine health information systems, will enable a public health-focused model of psychiatry based on collaborative working across specialties and sectors.

CONCLUSION

Global health has often been used as a euphemism for health problems in LMICs, but, as the case of mental health illustrates, problems with mental healthcare are truly global in nature. Mental health problems affect a wide section of the global population and, unfortunately, in what has been labelled as a 'failure of humanity', a large proportion of those affected are deprived of their basic human rights. Chronic neglect from policymakers and governmental and non-governmental funding agencies has led to a mental healthcare system starved of resources, especially of trained mental health professionals. The global problem currently is far too great for it to await the building up of capacity of mental health professionals, however, as at present levels of investment and training, this would take centuries rather than decades. Therefore, urgent systematic integration of mental health into the larger health system, strengthening public health programmes, PHC, education, social welfare and criminal justice programmes, is essential, from a human rights perspective and also from a physical health, educational, social and economic perspective.

REFERENCES

Crisp, A. (2004) 'The nature of stigmatisation' in A. Crisp (ed.), *Every Family in the Land: Understanding Prejudice and Discrimination against People with Mental Illness*. London: Royal Society of Medicine Press Ltd.

Gureje, O., Nortje, G., Makanjuola, V., Oladeji, B.D., Seedat, S. and Jenkins, R. (2015) 'The role of global traditional and complementary systems of medicine in the treatment of mental health disorders', *The Lancet Psychiatry*, 2 (2): 168–177.

Jenkins, R., Othieno, C., Okeyo, S., Kaseje, D., Aruwa, J., Oyugi, H. and Bassett, P. (2013) 'Short structured general mental health in service training programme in Kenya improves patient health and social outcomes but not detection of mental health problems: a pragmatic cluster randomised controlled trial', *International Journal of Mental Health Systems*, 7 (1): 25.

Lancet Mental Health Group (2007) 'Scale up services for mental disorders: a call for action', *The Lancet*, 370: 1241–1252.

Manderscheid, R. W., Ryff, C.D., McKight-Eily, L.R., Dhingra, S. and Strine, S.W. (2010) 'Evolving definitions of mental illness and wellness', *Preventing Chronic Disease*, 7(1): A19.

Patel, V. (2009) 'Integrating mental healthcare with chronic diseases in low-resource settings', *International Journal of Public Health*, 54: 1–3.

Saxena, S., Thornicroft, G., Knapp, M. and Whiteford, H. (2007) 'Resources for mental health: scarcity, inequity and inefficiency', *The Lancet*, 370: 878–889.

Thomas, P. and Bracken, P. (2004) 'Critical psychiatry in practice', *Advances in Psychiatric Practice*, 10: 361–370.

World Health Organization (n.d.) *Health Topics: Mental Health*. Available at: http://www.who.int/topics/mental_health/en (accessed 30 June 2015).

World Health Organization (2005) *Psychiatric Training Atlas*. Geneva: WHO.

World Health Organization (2006) *How Can the Human Rights of People with Mental Disorders be Promoted and Protected?* 5 October. Available at: www.who.int/features/qa/43/en/ (accessed 28 October 2013).

World Health Organization (2007) *What Is Mental Health?* 3 September. Available at: www.who.int/features/qa/62/en/index.html (accessed 26 October 2013).

World Health Organization (2011) *Mental Health Atlas*. Geneva: WHO.

12

MATERNAL HEALTH

DILEEP WIJERATNE AND ALISON FIANDER

Chapter overview

After reading this chapter you will be able to:

- describe factors affecting maternal health
- explain why human birth is a risky process
- explain how to reduce maternal mortality.

INTRODUCTION

Maternal health has improved over the past three decades. International data relating to maternal mortality suggests that the number of women who die annually has fallen from an estimated 530,000 in 1980 to just under 300,000 in 2011 (Lozano et al., 2011), as a result of collaboration between healthcare workers, policymakers, women's advocacy groups of individual countries and NGOs steered by the WHO and the MDGs. This has widened the availability of relatively inexpensive family planning, preventive and emergency medical interventions known for almost a century to reduce maternal mortality (Loudon, 2000).

Nevertheless, 300,000 deaths per year equates to more than 800 maternal deaths globally every day: one death every two minutes. Most of these deaths are due to causes for which treatments and/or prevention are well established, such as haemorrhage, sepsis, eclampsia and obstructed labour. Some 98 per cent of maternal deaths occur in LICs (UN, 2014). While the lifetime risk of death for a woman giving birth in Northern Europe is around 1 in 30,000, for a woman in parts of sub-Saharan Africa it is as high as 1 in 10 (Ronsmans and Graham, 2006). Maternal mortality remains the health statistic that shows the greatest disparity between HICs and LICs (WHO, 2014).

-------------------------------- Activity 12.1 --------------------------------

Search for the WHO's report *Trends in Maternal Mortality 1990–2013* (2014) on the Internet. Note the definition of maternal mortality and how it is measured.

Comment

A maternal death is, 'the death of a woman while pregnant or within 42 days of termination of pregnancy, irrespective of the duration and site of the pregnancy, from any cause related to or aggravated by the pregnancy or its management but not from accidental or incidental causes' (WHO, 2014: 4). The maternal mortality ratio (MMR) is the most commonly used measurement of maternal mortality and is also used as an MDG indicator. It is defined as the 'Number of maternal deaths during a given time period per 100,000 live births during the same time-period' (WHO, 2014: 6). MDG 5 – improving maternal health – had as its target to reduce the MMR by three quarters between 1990 and 2015. Globally, the overall combined MMR for all countries declined by 47 per cent between 1990 and 2010, from 400 to 210 (Lozano et al., 2011).

This chapter has three sections. Firstly, it looks at the nature of human pregnancy and birth from an anatomical and evolutionary perspective to understand why it is so dangerous in the first place. Then the specific interventions and health service characteristics that have reduced maternal mortality are described. Finally, implementation of these interventions in the context of highly variable global cultural, economic and social contexts is addressed.

WHY BIRTH IS DANGEROUS

Human pregnancy and birth are uniquely dangerous and complex because of the specific adaptations (or compromises) of human anatomy to accommodate our large brains and two-legged upright walking posture (Whitmann and Wall, 2007).

Thus, the female pelvis is comprised of several bones surrounding a central canal (the 'birth canal'), through which the baby passes during birth. The human pelvis has evolved to ensure that it can both support the entire upper body when upright and make walking and running on two legs as efficient as possible. To support the upper body, the top of the human pelvis is widest in the transverse diameter, providing plenty of stability and space for torso muscles to attach to. This means that the inlet of the human birth canal is widest in the transverse diameter. The bottom of the human pelvis, in contrast, is much narrower in the transverse diameter. This means that the human hip joints and legs are closer together, facilitating fast, efficient running and walking. The human birth canal is therefore widest at its outlet in the anterior-posterior (or front to back) diameter. The overall result is that the human birth canal is not a simple cylinder but, rather, a complex shape with a top that is widest in the transverse diameter and a bottom that is widest in the anterior-posterior diameter.

If the human foetus at the end of pregnancy had a head that was relatively small in comparison to the maternal pelvis, then even the complex shape of the human birth canal would not pose a significant problem. Human brains are large, however, to facilitate abilities such as complex language, fine motor skills and higher cognitive functions. As a result, in order to negotiate the birth canal, the foetal head must enter the pelvis in its widest (transverse) diameter, and then turn so that it exits the pelvis at its widest diameter (anterior-posterior).

In very general terms, the smallest diameter of the human foetal skull at the end of pregnancy is around 9.5cm. The average diameter of a female pelvic outlet is 10cm (Whitmann and Wall, 2007). So, if the foetal head adopts the wrong position fails to turn, if the pelvis is slightly too narrow, or if the uterine contractions are ineffective, birth will either take too long or not occur at all.

Many complications responsible for maternal mortality originate from the less than straightforward rotational birth mechanism going awry. If delivery takes too long, the uterus (womb) can become exhausted, significantly increasing the risk of post-partum haemorrhage. Dehydration and exhaustion occurring during a long labour also increase the risk of post-partum sepsis, especially when birth happens in an unclean environment. Without medical intervention, women can develop 'obstructed labour complex', whereby prolonged pressure on the placenta and umbilical cord often result in the death of the foetus. Also, prolonged pressure from the foetal head will eventually cause ischaemic necrosis of the soft tissues of the maternal pelvis, resulting in the formation of obstetric fistulae. These are abnormal communications that occur between the maternal bladder and/or rectum and the vagina, resulting in chronic incontinence of urine and/or faeces. Pressure on the pelvic nerves can result in conditions such as 'foot drop' and prolonged pressure on the muscles of the pelvic floor can result in severe utero-vaginal prolapse, either immediately or in later life. If the woman does not die from the obstructed labour itself, relief will only happen if she manages to either access medical care for a caesarean section or other instrumental delivery or if the baby dies, resulting in the eventual collapse of the foetal skull and vaginal delivery of a stillborn baby.

Globally, there are more than two million women and girls living with obstetric fistulae (WHO, 2014) and it is estimated that up to 100,000 new cases occur every year (Wall, 2006). Between 80 and 95 per cent of cases can be repaired surgically, but only if access to an appropriately trained person with adequate surgical facilities is available. Most women living with fistulae are unable to access treatment.

Activity 12.2

List the consequences of having an obstetric fistula under three categories – medical, psychological and social.

Comment

The medical consequences of obstetric fistulae include recurrent infection of the skin, genital tract and urinary tract, due to the chronic leakage of urine or faeces (or both). Such infections can in themselves be fatal or they can cause long-term severe consequences, such as chronic renal failure. Women living with fistulae experience high levels of divorce and social ostracism, with many left struggling to survive, with little support, on the margins of society. The end result of all this can be severe depression and, in the worst cases, even suicide (Murk, 2009).

The first steps towards reducing maternal mortality were seen in Europe in the 1750s when the essential features of the anatomy, physiology and pathology of childbirth were established, along with an improved understanding of how to manage the three stages of labour. The obstetric forceps, although invented a century earlier, also began to be used more widely to deal with obstructed labour. The first maternity hospitals were established in Europe, along with charities to provide antenatal support and midwifery attendance to the poor.

The eighteenth and nineteenth centuries also saw the emergence of midwifery as a profession, grounded in emerging scientific principles. In the UK, this culminated in the first Midwive's Act of 1902, regulating training in and practice of midwifery. The late 1800s also saw the widespread application of principles of antisepsis during delivery throughout Europe, which resulted in huge reductions in the number of women dying due to childbed fever (Loudon, 1992).

What is the evidence?

Childbed fever and maternal mortality

'Childbed fever' is the historical term used to describe what was, in the pre-antibiotic era, an often fatal infection acquired during or shortly after childbirth. Medical terms for this today are:

- chorioamnionitis – pre-delivery intrauterine sepsis
- endometritis – post-delivery intrauterine sepsis
- genital tract sepsis.

The most important organism with regard to childbed fever is Group A streptococcus, responsible for innumerable deaths over the centuries (Loudon, 2000). Globally, sepsis remains a significant contributor to maternal mortality and is still the commonest cause of death directly related to pregnancy.

The history of maternal care and antisepsis are intimately related. Ignaz Semmelweis noted that the rates of death due to childbed fever among women attended by medical students who had earlier in the day been performing autopsies were much higher than the rates among women attended by midwives only. His observances and ideas were not widely accepted and it was not until the principles of Listerian surgical antisepsis were widely applied to obstetric practice at the end of the nineteenth century that there was a major decline in deaths due to childbed fever. Prior to this, as many as one in ten women in the maternity hospitals of Europe may have died from childbed fever. The decline was further accelerated in the 1930s after the discovery of the sulphonamide and penicillin classes of antibiotics (Loudon, 1992).

Anaesthesia in childbirth gained popular acceptance when Queen Victoria used chloroform for the delivery of her eighth child in 1853. Further developments in anaesthesia in the twentieth century enabled obstetricians to perform caesarean sections safely. Improved blood transfusion technologies and antihaemorrhage drugs, such as ergometrine, developed during the first half of the twentieth century, also contributed to the decline in mortality. By the mid-1980s, there was a growing appreciation among the international community that most maternal deaths were preventable, even in low-resource settings (Rosenfield, 1985).

INTERVENTIONS FOR REDUCING MATERNAL MORTALITY IN LOW-RESOURCE SETTINGS

The global causes of maternal mortality are given in Table 12.1.

Table 12.1   Global causes of maternal mortality

Cause	Percentage
Combined Indirect Causes (e.g. Anaemia, Malaria, HIV, Heart disease)	28
Haemorrhage	27
Hypertension	14
Sepsis	11
Abortion	8
Embolism	3
Obstructed Labour and Other Direct Causes	9

Source: Adapted from Say et al. (2014)

Adapting the interventions developed in the industrialized world to country-specific contexts has enabled significant inroads to be made towards reducing maternal mortality in LMICs. The two most recent and high-profile international, multi-agency campaigns seeking to standardize this are the Safe Motherhood Initiative of 1987 and MDG 5.

Activity 12.3

List the targets for MDG 5.

THE SAFE MOTHERHOOD INITIATIVE

This established the 'four pillars of safe motherhood':

- family planning
- antenatal care
- clean and safe delivery
- essential obstetric care (EOC).

MDG 5

The specific targets are:

- **5A** Reduce by three quarters, between 1990 and 2015, the MMR
- **5B** Achieve, by 2015, universal access to reproductive health.

INTRAPARTUM CARE

Optimizing intrapartum care is the single most important intervention for reducing maternal mortality (Campbell and Graham, 2006), specifically through provision of skilled birth attendants, EOC and keeping the delivery as clean as possible. A basic level of EOC includes (WHO, 2009):

- parenteral antibiotics for management/prevention of sepsis
- drugs promoting uterine contraction and control of haemorrhage
- manual removal of retained placenta to prevent infection/haemorrhage (with adequate anaesthesia)
- removal of retained products of conception to prevent infection/haemorrhage
- administering of magnesium sulphate to women with eclampsia/pre-eclampsia
- performing assisted vaginal delivery by vacuum extraction/forceps
- performing basic neonatal resuscitation with a bag and mask.

In well-resourced HICs, most, if not all, of these procedures would be undertaken or at least directly supervised by a highly trained doctor. In LMICs, it is not unusual for basic EOC to be undertaken by midwives, nurses, physician assistants and, sometimes, traditional birth attendants.

The next step in intrapartum care is access to 'comprehensive' services, such as access to blood transfusion, medical ultrasound and surgical facilities for caesarean section and hysterectomy in cases of uncontrollable bleeding. The WHO cites a minimal caesarean delivery rate of 5 per cent as evidence of adequate access to these obstetric surgical services (WHO, 2001).

Where a maternal death is 'very rare', highly trained birth attendants (usually midwives) care for women, either in hospital or at home, and are able to detect and refer any complicated cases to secondary and tertiary facilities for assessment and treatment by obstetricians and other healthcare professionals. The World Bank and WHO have formally described the process through which countries' maternal health services develop with regard to EOC. This is a stepwise process, which progresses through four 'models' (Table 12.2).

Table 12.2   Provision of Essential Obstetric Care (EOC)

Model		Required factors of service delivery
1	Non-professional delivery at home	Non-professional recognizes complications
		Access to EOC arranged by non-professional or family, but functioning EOC is available
2	Skilled birth attendant delivery at home	As above but skilled attendant substituted for non-professional
3	Skilled birth attendant delivery in basic EOC facility (health centre)	Skilled attendant recognizes complications and provides basic EOC in health facility
		Basic EOC facility may organize transfer to functioning comprehensive facility if available
4	Skilled attendant delivery in comprehensive EOC facility (hospital)	Skilled attendant recognizes complications and provides basic and comprehensive emergency care

ANTENATAL CARE

Ideally intrapartum care should be supplemented by a robust antenatal care network, caring for women from the time of conception or early pregnancy in order to detect and manage complications of pregnancy early. Periodic measurement of blood pressure prevents up to 70 per cent of eclampsia cases by detecting pre-eclampsia early. The WHO recommends providing a minimum of four antenatal care visits, where women contact a trained healthcare professional – either a midwife or a doctor (WHO, 2014). As of 2012, globally, only 52 per cent of pregnant women had four or more antenatal care visits, although this represents a significant increase from a figure of just 37 per cent in 1990 (UN, 2014).

In LMICs, the antenatal visits should include:

- tetanus toxoid vaccination
- checking for anaemia
- identifying warning signs, such as increasing blood pressure
- screening and treatment for infections, such as syphilis and HIV.

In countries where malaria is endemic, pregnant women should also receive close monitoring, with intermittent treatment if required, to prevent/treat the disease and reduce adverse outcomes for mother and baby. Pregnant women who test positive for HIV should receive medication and advice to help prevent maternal fetal transmission of infection.

Activity 12.4

List the benefits to mother and baby of treating HIV during pregnancy.

Comment

In 2013, the WHO recommended triple antiviral therapy for all pregnant women with HIV. Treatment has significantly reduced maternal mortality from infections such as endometritis, pneumonia, TB and malaria. A systematic review showed that, in the absence of HIV, there would have been 60,000 fewer maternal deaths in 2008 alone (Hogan et al., 2010). Without treatment, the risk of perinatal transmission of HIV from mother to baby varies between 15 and 45 per cent, depending on the mode of delivery and maternal viral levels at delivery, which can be reduced by treating the mother. With effective interventions, this rate can be reduced to levels below 5 per cent.

In HICs with good access to clean water and high-quality formula feeds, breastfeeding by mothers with HIV is often discouraged. In LMICs, the risks of ingesting unclean water and poor-quality formula often outweigh the risks of viral transmission via breastfeeding. The WHO recommends that all infants born to a HIV+ mother receive post-exposure antiretroviral prophylaxis for six weeks after birth. A longer duration may be warranted if the infant is breastfeeding and his or her mother did not receive antiretroviral agents prior to labour. The WHO recommends a minimum of at least six months of exclusive breastfeeding, along with antiviral treatment given to the mother (with or without antiretrovirals for the baby, depending on the clinical scenario).

Read and note the WHO's *Consolidated Guidelines on the Use of Antiretroviral Drugs for Treating and Preventing HIV Infection* (2013).

A comprehensive antenatal care system provides:

- services where antenatal care is accessible to all women, irrespective of geographical location and socio-economic status, with outreach services to rural regions with poor transport links and free or heavily subsidized services for the poorest women
- nationally agreed standards and protocols for the management of both normal and complicated pregnancies
- access to skilled health professionals and essential medicines
- service linkage to a healthcare system to provide continuity of care in the post-partum period
- adequate recording and reporting systems and use of data to improve the quality of care
- policies addressing social and cultural barriers to care.

FAMILY PLANNING

By 2015, it is projected that population growth will increase the global demand for family planning among married women alone to almost one billion, demonstrating the scale of the efforts needed to meet the demand for contraceptives, especially the more effective modern methods, especially LARCs. For non-pregnant women, access to contraception contributes cost-effectively to a reduction in maternal mortality (UN, 2014). The provision of contraception saves lives through its reduction of unwanted pregnancies, which, in turn:

- decreases pregnancy-related mortality
- decreases abortion-related mortality
- delays first pregnancy in adolescents whose incomplete pelvic development increases the risk of obstructed labour
- reduces the total number of children a woman has – increasing parity increases the risk of placenta praevia and post-partum haemorrhage
- reduces the risk of early pregnancy complications (such as miscarriage and ectopic pregnancy)
- reduces closely spaced pregnancies, so mothers recover between pregnancies.

In 2005, the global death toll due to unsafe abortion was estimated to be around 70,000, which is 1 in 8 of all maternal deaths. Almost all of these deaths occurred in LMICs. Sociocultural and religious stigma impede the provision of safe abortion services in many places, making pregnancy prevention through effective contraception vital. In regions such as most of Northern Europe and China, where clean, safe and non-restricted abortion services are available (usually free of charge), carried out by skilled healthcare professionals, maternal deaths related to abortion are rare.

PROGRESS TOWARDS MDG 5

In 2000, the stated aim of MDG 5A was to reduce the MMR by three quarters between 1990 and 2015, by reducing the number of deaths in countries where the MMR was raised. The main focus, therefore, was on countries where the MMR was raised (>100), high (>300) or very high (>1000).

Although the maternal mortality targets of MDG 5 have not been met in their entirety, there has still been remarkable progress. Globally, the MMR declined by 47 per cent between 1990 and 2013, from 400 to 210 maternal deaths per 100,000 live births. All regions of the world have made progress, with the highest reductions being seen in Eastern Asia (69 per cent), Northern Africa (66 per cent) and Southern Asia (64 per cent; WHO, 2014). In spite of these encouraging figures, out of all the MDGs, it is the target of MDG 5 towards which the least amount of progress has been made (UN, 2014).

Countries making significant progress demonstrate:

- effective leadership, with political will prioritizing maternal health, ideally at every level
- effective partnership working
- effective application of context-sensitive medical and public health evidence of maternal health
- both short- and long-term strategies
- responsiveness to socio-economic change
- policies grounded in human rights
- improving the availability and quality of regional and national maternal death audits, as this contributes to better estimates of maternal mortality, while also helping to initiate the taking of actions necessary to prevent future deaths.

The aim of MDG 5B was to achieve, by 2015, universal access to reproductive health (such as ensuring access to contraceptive services). The unmet need for family planning – defined as the percentage of women aged 15 to 49, married or in a sexually active relationship, who report the desire to delay or avoid pregnancy but who are not using any form of contraception – has declined from 17 per cent in 1990 to 12 per cent in the most recent global estimate from 2012. The current shortfall translates into around 140 million women worldwide who would like to delay or avoid pregnancy, but are unable to access effective contraception (UN, 2014). Thus, in spite of significant progress, universal access to reproductive health is still some way off.

BARRIERS TO REDUCING MATERNAL MORTALITY

Every place where maternal mortality is high has its own unique set of economic, financial, cultural, geographical and social conditions. Poor transport infrastructure can prevent women from accessing care, although simple innovations such as cycle ambulances may reduce transfer delays. Other factors include:

- financial constraints
- conflict
- gender inequality.

Evidence from around the world demonstrates that measures to reduce gender inequality, coupled with programmes to reduce maternal mortality, are highly effective. For example, maternal mortality has fallen by 75 per cent in two indigenous communities in La Paz, Bolivia, where women's groups have implemented education and empowerment programmes, educated men about gender equality and reproductive health and trained community health workers (UN, 2014). In contrast, those countries in the world with the highest rates of maternal mortality, such as Sierra Leone, Niger and the Democratic Republic of Congo, also have the lowest scores in composite measures of gender equality.

CONCLUSION

From the discussions in this chapter we can see that a maternal death is never an isolated event and will always be embedded in a complex network of biological, cultural, political and socio-economic causal factors. An appreciation of this complexity is a crucial prerequisite when designing effective maternal health programmes.

We have also seen that the specific medical interventions, characteristics of health systems and even social conditions necessary to reduce maternal mortality are being understood in increasingly rich levels of nuance and detail. One of the major challenges of the post-2015 era will be how to apply and build on our knowledge of combating maternal mortality to ensure that access to effective reproductive healthcare services for all of world's most vulnerable women and girls. If this challenge is met and the momentum for improvement of the past three decades is sustained, then the UN has predicted that preventable maternal mortality is a scourge that can be ended, across the globe, within a generation.

REFERENCES

Campbell, O. and Graham, W.J. (2006) 'Strategies for reducing maternal mortality: getting on with what works', *The Lancet*, 368(9543): 1284–1299.

Hogan, M.C., Foreman K.J., Naghavi, M., Ahn, S.Y., Wang, M., Makela, S.M. et.al. (2010) 'Maternal mortality for 181 countries, 1980–2008: a systematic analysis of progress towards Millennium Development Goal 5', *The Lancet*, 375(9726): 1609–1623.

Loudon, I. (1992) 'The transformation of maternal mortality', *British Medical Journal*, 368(6868): 1557–1560.

Loudon, I. (2000) 'Maternal mortality in the past and its relevance to developing countries today', *The American Journal of Clinical Nutrition*, 72(1): 241–246.

Lozano, R., Wang, H., Foreman, K.J., Rajaratnam, J.K., Naghavi, M., Marcus, J.R. et al. (2011) 'Progress towards Millennium Development Goals 4 and 5 on maternal and child mortality: an updated systematic analysis', *The Lancet*, 378(9797): 1139–1165.

Murk, W. (2009) 'Experiences with Obstetric Fistula in rural Uganda', *The Yale Journal of Biology and Medicine*, 82(2): 79–82.

Ronsmans, C. and Graham, W.J. (2006) 'Maternal mortality: who, when, where, and why', *The Lancet*, 368(9542): p1189.

Rosenfield, A. (1985) 'Maternal mortality – a neglected tragedy: where is the M in MCH?', *The Lancet*, 13(8446): 83–85.

Say, L., Chou, D., Gemmill, A., Tunçalp, O., Moller, A., Daniels, J. et al. (2014) 'Global causes of maternal death: a WHO systematic analysis', *Lancet Glob Health*, 2: e323–33.

United Nations (2014) *Millennium Development Goal Report 2014*. New York: United Nations.

Wall, L. (2006) 'Obstetric vesicovaginal fistula as an international public-health problem', *The Lancet*, 368(9542): 1201–1209.

Wittman, A. and Wall, L. (2007) 'The evolutionary origins of obstructed labor: bipedalism, encephalization, and the human obstetric dilemma', *Obstet Gynecol Surv*, 62(11): 739–748.

WHO (2001) 'Maternal mortality at the end of a decade: signs of progress?', *Bulletin of the World Health Organization*, 79(6): 561.

WHO (2009) *Monitoring Emergency Obstetric Care: A Handbook*. Geneva: World Health Organization.

WHO (2013) *Consolidated Guidelines on the Use of Antiretroviral Drugs for Treating and Preventing HIV Infection*. Geneva: WHO.

WHO (2014) *Trends in Maternal Mortality 1990–2013*. Geneva: World Health Organization.

13

CHILD AND ADOLESCENT HEALTH

BHANU WILLIAMS, ANU GOENKA, DAN MAGNUS AND STEPHEN ALLEN

Chapter overview

After reading this chapter you should be able to describe, in the context of child and adolescent health and well-being:

- the MDGs
- disease burden at the global level and common causes of death
- important socio-economic, cultural, educational and environmental determinants
- interventions available to combat the major threats to health and well-being
- approaches to child protection and setting priorities.

THE MDGS – DRIVING THE GLOBAL HEALTH AGENDA

In September 2000, the leaders of 192 UN member states adopted the Millennium Declaration. Using 1990 as a baseline, eight MDGs bound countries to halve severe poverty, widespread hunger and illiteracy and reduce environmental deterioration and discrimination against women by 2015. Many of the MDGs included in their targets specific, measurable indicators for both children and adolescents (see Table 13.1).

Table 13.1 MDG indicators specific to children and adolescents

MDGs	Indicator
Goal 1 Eradicate extreme poverty and hunger	Prevalence of underweight children under five years of age.
Goal 2 Achieve universal primary education	Net enrolment ratio in primary education.
	Proportion of pupils starting grade 1 who reach grade 5.
	Literacy rate of 15–24-year-olds.

MDGs	Indicator
Goal 3 Promote gender equality and empower women	Ratio of girls to boys in primary, secondary and tertiary education.
	Ratio of literate women to men at 15–24 years old.
Goal 4 Reduce child mortality	Under-five mortality rate (per 1000 live births).
	Infant mortality rate (per 1000 live births).
	Proportion of one-year-old children immunized against measles.
Goal 6 Combat HIV/AIDS, malaria and other diseases	Prevalence of HIV among pregnant women 15–24 years old.
	Percentage of population aged 15–24 years with comprehensive correct knowledge of HIV/AIDS.
	Ratio of school attendance of orphans to school attendance of non-orphans aged 10–14 years.
Goal 8 Global partnership for development	Unemployment rate of young people aged 15–24 years, each sex and total.

Source: Adapted from the information on MDGs available from the UN's Millennium Project website (at: www.unmillenniumproject.org/goals/gti.htm).

The MDGs have contributed to a concerted international effort to improve health and well-being among the world's poorest people and remarkable progress has been made in many countries.

─────────────── Activity 13.1 ───────────────

Write down your answers to the following questions.

1. Globally, how many children die below their fifth birthday?
2. What are the big killers?
3. What proportion of deaths of children under the age of five years occur in the neonatal period?
4. How do mortality rates of children under the age of five years vary across different countries?

Comment

Regarding MDG 4, under-five mortality (UFM – that is, deaths below the age of five years per 1000 live births) has fallen by about half – from 90 in 1990 (12.6 million deaths) to 48 per 1000 (6.6 million) in 2012 (UNICEF, 2013). The biggest killers are pneumonia, diarrhoeal diseases and malaria and 44 per cent of UFM occurs in the neonatal period.

Even with rising population size, UFM has declined in all regions and the MDG 4 goal has already been reached in some. Among the 61 high-mortality countries (UFM of ≥ 40), UFM between 1990 and 2012 has fallen by at least half in 25 countries and by two-thirds or more in seven. Progress in sub-Saharan Africa, however, is slower, which means that half of all such child deaths now occur in this region. All of the 16 countries with UFM of >100 are in sub-Saharan Africa.

The slowest declines in UFM have occurred in West and Central Africa so that, combined with a rising under-five population, the total number of child deaths in these regions has remained fairly constant. In terms of absolute numbers of deaths, high mortality rates combine with large population size so that half of all child deaths occur in just five countries: India (22 per cent), Nigeria (13 per cent), Pakistan (6 per cent), the Democratic Republic of Congo (6 per cent) and China (4 per cent).

INEQUITY IN CHILD DEATHS

There is marked inequity in child mortality between countries. In 2012, average UFM in LICs (82/1000 live births) was more than 13 times higher than in HICs. The country estimated to have the highest UFM rate was Sierra Leone (182/1000 live births) and the lowest rates occurred in Iceland and Luxembourg (2/1000 live births (UNICEF, 2013).

In addition to differences between countries, marked inequalities in health also occur within countries, reflecting multiple disadvantages in marginalized groups, including poor access to healthcare. The assessment of the coverage of life-saving interventions according to the economic status of the population now provides critical information for designing effective interventions specific to local contexts.

WHAT ARE THE MAJOR DISEASES CAUSING CHILD DEATHS?

Table 13.2 shows the global causes of child deaths in 2013 broken down by those occurring within and outside the neonatal period (0–28 days).

Table 13.2   Major causes of child deaths in 2013

	Pre-term birth complications	15 per cent
	Intrapartum-related events	11 per cent
	Sepsis or meningitis	7 per cent
Child deaths in neonatal period	Congenital abnormalities	4 per cent
(44 per cent)	Other neonatal disorders	4 per cent
	Tetanus	1 per cent
	Pneumonia	2 per cent
	Pneumonia	13 per cent
	Diarrhoea	9 per cent
	Malaria	7 per cent
	Injury	5 per cent
Child deaths outside of neonatal period	Measles	2 per cent
(56 per cent)	AIDS	2 per cent
	Meningitis	2 per cent
	Pertussis	2 per cent
	Other disorders	14 per cent

Source: Adapted from Liu et al. (2015)

THE NEONATAL PERIOD

The decline in death rates in the neonatal period has been slower than for older children. At present, deaths during this period account for 44 per cent of all child deaths (2.9 million each year) with complications during delivery and consequent birth asphyxia and pre-term births being the major contributors (Martines et al., 2005; see also Chapter 12). About one million deaths occur on the first day of life and more than two in three of these deaths are preventable, even with limited resources (Darmstadt, 2005). See Table 13.3.

Table 13.3   Interventions to improve neonatal survival

Antenatal	Intrapartum	Postnatal
• Tetanus toxoid immunization	• Antibiotics for prolonged rupture of membranes	• Newborn resuscitation
• Syphilis screening	• Steroids in pre-term labour	• Breastfeeding
• Pre-eclampsia management	• Management of breech presentation	• Kangaroo Mother Care
• Intermittent presumptive treatment of malaria	• Use of partogram	• Postnatal community visits
• Treatment of asymptomatic bacteriuria	• Clean delivery practices	

Source: Martines et al. (2005)

The challenges in providing a comprehensive package of interventions was highlighted by an evaluation of the WHO's Essential Newborn Care Course, which failed to demonstrate a significant decrease in perinatal mortality, but did demonstrate a decrease in the rate of stillbirths. Evidence from Rwanda highlighted the need to regularly update skills taught in the Helping Babies Breathe programme, which focuses on newborn resuscitation. Although some neonatal interventions have been adapted for use in low-resource settings, such as bubble nasal continuous positive airways pressure for respiratory distress syndrome of prematurity, the evidence base for the efficacy of most interventions is poor, indicating an urgent need for high-quality randomized trials.

DIARRHOEA AND PNEUMONIA – THE BIG KILLERS

Diarrhoea and pneumonia are the leading causes of death in older infants and children (13 per cent and 8 per cent of child deaths in 2012, respectively), especially in children under two years old. The two causes are linked together because the underlying risk factors (undernutrition, poor hygiene, suboptimal breastfeeding, zinc deficiency) and effective interventions (access to safe water, improved sanitation) overlap (Walker et al., 2013). This has encouraged the development of integrated programmes to prevent both diseases.

Mortality from diarrhoeal disease is decreasing, but many deaths remain preventable. A recent multicentre study confirmed rotavirus as the leading cause of moderate–severe diarrhoea in children. A rotavirus vaccine has already been introduced in 45 countries and the Gavi Alliance (global Vaccine Alliance) plans to make it available to all developing countries (Bhutta et al., 2013).

Integrated Management of Childhood Illness (IMCI) case definitions have helped simplify the classification of diarrhoea syndromes (acute, persistent, bloody), as well as dehydration severity (none, some and severe). Treatment is based on oral rehydration solution and early refeeding. Oral zinc administration reduces both the severity and duration of diarrhoea and prevents subsequent episodes.

Activity 13.2

Search on the Internet for research on the effectiveness of Hib vaccines.

Comment

Perhaps you came across the systematic review by Jackson et al. (2012) 'Systematic review of observational data on effectiveness of *Haemophilus influenzae* type b (Hib) vaccines to allow optimization of vaccination schedules' (at: www.who.int/immunization/sage/meetings/2012/november/4._Systematic_review_of_observational_data_on_effectiveness_of_Hib_vaccines_Jackson_C_et_al_2012.pdf).

Deaths from the two leading causes of pneumonia, *Haemophilus influenzae* type b (Hib) and *Streptococcus pneumoniae*, have reduced as a result of Hib vaccines having been introduced in 184 countries and pneumococcal conjugate vaccines (PCV) in 88 countries. Unexpected benefits of PCV were demonstrated in South Africa, emphasizing the overall importance of pneumococcal infection. Outcomes were also improved in children with viral pneumonia and those without chest X-ray changes.

WHO guidelines have simplified pneumonia classification into 'non-severe' and 'severe', according to the level of respiratory distress. There remains a problem with education at the community level, however, with only 60 per cent of children with a cough and difficulty breathing seeking healthcare (UNICEF, 2013). Despite the limited specificity of WHO case definitions, their use within the IMCI strategy has reduced mortality by up to 20 per cent in some settings. The improved detection of hypoxaemia and treatment with oxygen concentrators has also been shown to be associated with a 35 per cent reduction in pneumonia mortality. Access to appropriate antibiotic therapy is essential to avoid sepsis and the necessity for fluid resuscitation, with careful prescribing to deter the development of antibiotic resistance.

What is the evidence?

The Fluid Expansion as Supportive Therapy (FEAST) trial (Maitland et al., 2011) was conducted in several African centres without ventilation facilities and 3000 children with fever and impaired circulation were randomly assigned to receive either intravenous fluid bolus or no bolus.

The study was halted prematurely as interim analyses demonstrated increased mortality at 48 hours in the fluid bolus group (relative risk 1.45; 95 per cent confidence interval:

1.13 to 1.86). Debate over the findings has centred on the study's definition of shock, which some critics argue was inadequate and not the same as that used by the WHO. Nevertheless, some experts are now advocating increased caution in administering intravenous fluids to febrile children with impaired circulation.

MALARIA

There has been great progress in reducing morbidity and mortality from malaria with a focus on prevention and treatment of *Plasmodium falciparum*, the species responsible for severe malaria. Long-lasting insecticide-treated bed nets (ITNs) substantially reduce the vector population of *Anopheles* mosquitoes and the incidence of malaria. The WHO now recommends the universal use of ITNs in regions where malaria is endemic, including for school-age children. Almost 40 per cent of children in sub-Saharan African countries use ITNs, but usage varies considerably, both between and within countries (UNICEF, 2013).

Syndromic clinical diagnostic approaches to malaria without laboratory confirmation of infection are unspecific and fuel drug resistance through the inappropriate treatment of non-malarial fever. Access to diagnostic tests for malaria for children with fever remains low with marked inequity in access to care in some countries. Thus, rapid diagnostic tests (RDTs) have been developed for patients' use and are cost-effective. Also, the artemesinin derivatives are safe and rapidly acting anti-malarials prevent malaria transmission by killing gametocytes. In a concerted effort to delay drug resistance, the artemesinins are formulated as combination therapy (ACT) so that the partner drugs kill any artemesinin-resistant parasites. ACT is now the cornerstone of malaria treatment and is recommended in the majority of countries where malaria is endemic. Rectal artesunate may be an important and accessible alternative to injectable forms for children without rapid access to health facilities. Of concern is that artemisinin resistance has emerged in South East Asia, highlighting the need for integrated programmes combining vector control with RDT/ACT rollout and the development of an effective vaccine.

What is the evidence?

AQUAMAT was a large African multicentre trial carried out from 2005 until 2010 involving over 5000 children with severe malaria who were randomized to receive treatment with intravenous quinine or artesunate (Dondorp et al., 2010). Artesunate was associated with reduced mortality (there was a risk reduction of 22.5 per cent, with a 95 per cent confidence interval 8.1–36.9), as well as reduced coma and convulsions, when compared with quinine.

UNDERNUTRITION

Global estimates of undernutrition in children are striking. In 2012, an estimated 51 million children suffered from wasting, with 80 per cent living in either south Asia or sub-Saharan Africa, while 162 million had moderate or severe stunting

(UNICEF, 2013). Obesity poses additional burdens in LICs as well as MICs and HICs. Undernutrition is an underlying factor in 45 per cent of deaths in children under the age of five (about three million deaths per year) through increasing susceptibility to and mortality from infections such as pneumonia (UNICEF, 2013). Because of its high prevalence, moderate rather than severe undernutrition underlies the majority of undernutrition-associated deaths. In addition, the detrimental effects on school performance and cognitive development have been well documented. Growth failure occurring in the first two years of life may result in irreversible long-term short stature. The 'first 1000 days', including the period from conception, have been highlighted as a major target for nutrition interventions.

Undernutrition is usually multifactorial and exacerbated by civil conflict, drought, flooding and other effects of climate change on vulnerable populations. Prevention focuses on improving the coverage of key interventions, such as breastfeeding, complementary feeding and micronutrient supplements, including vitamin A. Undernutrition in schoolchildren is particularly common in Africa, where stunting (prevalence 8.8 per cent to 52.5 per cent) and wasting (13.7 per cent to 15.6 per cent) in children aged between four-and-a-half and 18 years is common, especially in boys and older school-age children. School feeding programmes improve weight gain by between 0.25 and 0.75 kilograms per year, gender equity in access to education, school attendance and cognition and school performance.

Children with severe acute malnutrition (SAM) present a huge challenge to under-resourced health facilities. There are wide variations in inpatient mortality rates, which, in part, can be explained by variations in leadership, supervision and teamwork. The WHO case definitions to identify SAM have been simplified and include mid-upper arm circumference (MUAC), which can be performed in any setting. Complicated undernutrition requires admission to hospital or a specialist feeding centre for implementation of the WHO's 10 Steps to Recovery. The management of SAM that is uncomplicated (there is no fever or anorexia, for example) should be undertaken in the community, incorporating the use of ready-to-use therapeutic foods.

HIV AND AIDS

About 1.5 million pregnant girls and women (aged 15 and above) are living with HIV, 90 per cent of whom are in sub-Saharan Africa (UNICEF, 2013). Globally, the rate of new perinatal HIV infections is decreasing, largely because of the success of the prevention of mother-to-child transmission (PMTCT) programmes. The WHO now advocates lifelong antiretroviral therapy (ART) for all pregnant women and all HIV-infected children under five years old, irrespective of CD4 count, though some national guidelines have not yet incorporated this guidance.

A trial demonstrated that early initiation of ART in infancy resulted in a 75 per cent reduction in mortality and progression of the disease compared with deferred treatment (Violari, 2008). In 2011, however, only 23 per cent of eligible HIV-infected children were receiving ART. Other trials have demonstrated that ART without laboratory monitoring was safe and effective in HIV-infected children from Zimbabwe and Uganda.

NEGLECTED ISSUES

ADOLESCENT HEALTH

Historically, the health of adolescents (defined by the WHO as young people between 10 and 19 years of age) has received much less attention than that of younger children, despite the importance of adolescence as the foundation of adult health. Several measurable targets for the health of young people aged from 15 to 24 years were, however, included in the MDGs (see Table 13.1, earlier in this chapter).

The leading causes of death in adolescence are injuries (both road traffic accidents and suicide) and maternal causes. Access to education and national wealth are the strongest determinants of adolescent health and supportive families, schools and peers are needed to ensure the best health outcomes. Programmes specifically targeting adolescents and better data on adolescent outcomes are also priorities.

Among the non-fatal illnesses, the largest disease burden in adolescence is due to mental illness, with 75 per cent of all mental health disorders being recognized first in this age group. Mental health disorders are closely correlated with substance abuse and poorer educational attainment (see Chapter 11). Additional risk factors include a family history of mental illness, prenatal exposure to toxins, under-nutrition, HIV infection, maltreatment as a child, poverty and unsupportive family, school and community backgrounds.

There are difficulties in obtaining reliable data on the burden of mental disorders in adolescence, particularly in LICs, but the available data point to suicide as a leading cause of death of young people in India and China (see Chapter 10). Child and adolescent mental health policies are deficient in African and South East Asian countries compared with richer nations. Timely access to drug and psychotherapy support for young people is inadequate in well-resourced countries and even worse in poorer countries. Mental health interventions for young people need to be included in existing health and education programmes.

CHILD PROTECTION

The maltreatment of children remains a global public health problem, but almost all the available data on the burden, recognition and effectiveness of interventions originates from HICs.

Maltreatment is usually classified as neglect, physical, mental or sexual abuse or a combination thereof. Professionals working in different settings may experience difficulties with different cultural norms relating to the physical punishment of children, child labour and female genital mutilation. The role of poverty in neglect may be particularly difficult as abusive intent may be difficult to establish. The physical health consequences of child maltreatment and neglect, such as burns or sexually transmitted infections, are likely to be easier to manage than the psychosocial effects.

Professionals should work within multidisciplinary teams and harness local knowledge to promote a child's best interests. The UN Convention on the Rights of the Child extends beyond protection to the right of a child to receive education and participation in decisions affecting children (UNICEF, 2013).

HELMINTH INFECTIONS AND DEWORMING

Around one billion children live in areas where soil-transmitted helminth infection is endemic. Worm infections are most common in school-age children and they account for 20 per cent of DALYs lost due to communicable diseases in these children. Studies have shown associations between helminth infections and undernutrition, anaemia, poor growth and school attendance and poor performance in cognition tests.

Although the World Bank and WHO promote helminth control programmes in LMIC settings as a cost-effective intervention, the benefits are unclear. A single dose of deworming drugs in children with confirmed infection results in a small increase in weight (0.58 kg) and haemoglobin of (0.37 g/dL), but its effectiveness when administered to all children in regions where such infections are endemic is uncertain.

Activity 13.3

Search for 'Turkana and hydatid disease' on the Internet. Make a note of the role of cultural factors in the transmission of the disease.

Comment

Among the Turkana pastoralists of northern Kenya, there was a high prevalence of hydatid disease (of between 5 and 10 per cent), which led the medical charity African Medical Research Foundation (AMREF) to introduce a control programme.

Epidemiological studies there showed dogs and jackals to be the main definitive hosts of *Echinococcus granulosus* (Nelson, 1986). This parasite significantly reduces meat and milk production, as well as causing fertility loss in livestock. It is also one of the major zoonotic parasitic diseases afflicting humans.

Were you surprised to find out that Turkana dogs serve as nursemaids to children who have yet to be toilet-trained and lick clean infants after they vomit? While there are now few incident cases in the under-five population, the programme was not as effective as was anticipated because of the nomadic traditions and the close affinity the Turkana people have with their dogs.

PREVENTION OF TRAUMA AND/OR ACCIDENTS

Violence and injury are significant threats globally to child health, but more than 95 per cent of all injury deaths in children occur in LMICs. Around 950,000 deaths per year under the age of 18 years are attributable to trauma/injury (WHO, 2008). Some 90 per cent of these are unintentional, but they are the leading cause of death for children aged 10 to 19 years. In all age groups, the leading causes of death and injury are road traffic accidents, drowning and fire-related burns. Road traffic accidents alone are the leading cause of death in children aged 15 to 19 years and they are the second leading cause among 10- to 14-year-olds. It is also important to remember the many millions of children who require hospital care each year for non-fatal injuries, many of which may result in permanent disability.

WIDER DETERMINANTS OF CHILD AND ADOLESCENT HEALTH

SOCIO-ECONOMIC STATUS, FOOD SECURITY AND MATERNAL EDUCATION

Poor food security and low socio-economic status with limited access to resources are a precursor for malnutrition and poor growth and development in children. Demographic and health surveys in Kenya have indicated that place of residence, level of wealth, type of drinking water and toilet access impact undernutrition. The poorest children are more likely to be stunted, wasted and underweight than the richest. Protective factors include longer duration of breastfeeding, higher maternal age at first birth and up-to-date vaccination status.

Improvements in female education are estimated to have resulted in more than half of the decline in UFM (UNICEF, 2013). Improved maternal education protects against undernutrition and is associated with improved child vaccination status, delayed marriage and childbirth. At the country level, there is a very close association between level of female education and UFM.

URBAN THREATS IN AN URBANIZING WORLD

UNICEF predicts that by 2050 seven in ten people will live in urban areas, with an annual increase in urban populations of around 60 million people, predominantly occurring in LMICs.

--- **Activity 13.4** ---

Write down countries where you think most of the urban growth is taking place.

Comment

Half of the world's urban population lives in Asia and, of the 100 fastest-growing areas, 33 are in China. Rates of urbanization are slower in Africa, but 60 per cent of urban dwellers in Africa live in slums. Much of the urbanization in LICs is not taking place in 'megacities', but in smaller cities and towns where the majority of urban children can be found.

On average, children in urban areas are more likely to survive infancy and early childhood, enjoy better health and nutritional status and have more educational opportunities than their counterparts in rural areas. This effect is often referred to as the 'urban advantage'.

Although there are some benefits, poor urban children remain at risk of non-communicable diseases, abuse of alcohol, tobacco and drugs, threats posed to mental health and poor nutrition, including obesity, and injuries. Living in slums in particular poses many problems for children. The UN's Human Settlements Programme defines a household in a slum as one that lacks one or more of the following:

- access to improved water
- access to improved sanitation
- security of tenure
- durability of housing
- sufficient living area.

Gaps between rich and poor within towns and cities can sometimes equal or exceed those found in rural areas. Many children living in urban poverty are excluded from higher education, health services and other benefits enjoyed by their more affluent peers. Although there is much inequality in rural areas, urban poverty can also profoundly limit educational opportunities for children. Some disparities transcend location, however – girls growing up in poor households are at a great disadvantage, regardless of whether they live in urban or rural areas.

VACCINATION AND THE EXPANDED PROGRAMME ON IMMUNIZATION (EPI)

Although immunization currently averts an estimated two to three million deaths every year, it is estimated that 1.5 million children died globally in 2010 from vaccine-preventable diseases, for which there were WHO prequalified vaccines available.

The EPI was established in 1974, as a result of a World Health Assembly resolution to build on the success of the global smallpox eradication programme. Through collaboration between the WHO and the global Vaccine Alliance (Gavi Alliance), the EPI has been successfully developed, such that, in 2012, more than 80 per cent of infants were vaccinated against diphtheria, tuberculosis, pertussis, polio, measles and tetanus (UNICEF, 2013).

Additional vaccines have now been added to the original six recommended in 1974. As detailed above, more countries, including the majority of LICs, are adding hepatitis B, Hib, PCV and rotavirus vaccines to their routine infant immunization schedules. Despite the huge success of the EPI, it is worth remembering, however, that, in 2010, approximately 19.3 million children did not receive even the DTP3 vaccinations worldwide, with more than a third of these children living in Africa.

Case study   The EPI and Malawi

Malawi has a total population of 16 million. In 1990, it had the second-highest mortality rate for children under the age of five years (UFM) in southern and eastern Africa. In contrast to many of its neighbours, however, Malawi has seen a substantial decline in its UFM from 244 in every 1000 live births in 1990 to 71 in 2012. These improvements have been in no small part due to the effective roll-out of the EPI. Overall, DTP3 coverage was 96 per cent in 2013, with all districts achieving at least 80 per cent DTP3 vaccine coverage. Malawi has also introduced pneumococcal and rotavirus vaccines, alongside BCG, DTP3, measles, hepatitis B and Hib vaccines.

WATER, SANITATION AND HYGIENE

Unsafe water, poor sanitation and unhygienic conditions are still a significant problem for children around the world. These factors underlie deaths from acute diarrhoea and pneumonia. In addition, persistent diarrhoea (≥14 days duration) contributes to undernutrition and reduced resistance to infections. An estimated 770 million people do not use an improved source for drinking water, including 185 million who rely on surface water to meet their daily drinking water needs. By the end of 2011, 83 per cent of the population without access to improved drinking water lived in rural areas. Although only 4 per cent of the urban population relies on unimproved sources, supplies are often intermittent, increasing contamination risks. In urban slums, insufficient water supply and sanitation combine with over-crowded conditions to maximize faecal contamination and increase the risks of diarrhoea and other infections.

Globally, around 2.5 billion people lack access to an improved sanitation facility. Of these, 761 million use public or shared sanitation facilities and another 693 million use facilities that do not meet minimum standards of hygiene. Open defecation is practised by the remaining one billion. The majority (71 per cent) of those without sanitation live in rural areas, where 90 per cent of all open defecation takes place. Urban populations tend to have better access to sanitation than rural populations, but, as a result of rapid urban population growth, the number of urban dwellers practising open defecation increased from 140 million to 169 million between 1990 and 2008.

Activity 13.5

List a behavioural change that would reduce the risk of infection in the circumstances just described.

Comment

Hand washing with soap has been advocated as one of the most effective interventions for improving child nutrition and survival. Hand washing interrupts the faecal–oral transmission route of pathogens and resulted in a 31 per cent reduction in diarrhoeal episodes when prac-tised in LMICs. A randomized controlled trial of hand washing in Pakistan also demonstrated a reduction in the incidence of pneumonia by 50 per cent and impetigo by 34 per cent. No difference has been shown between normal and antibacterial soaps (Luby et al., 2005).

GETTING INVOLVED IN GLOBAL CHILD HEALTH

There are many opportunities for healthcare workers to contribute to global child health. They can build on skills they have already acquired, as well as make a valuable contribution to a health system in another country or region. Placements can be organized through established programmes or on a more ad hoc basis through direct communication with host institutions. In the USA, 70 per cent of paediatric residency programmes incorporate global child health components. This usually consists of a placement in a low-resource setting for either clinical work or research.

A vast number of non-governmental organizations (NGOs) cater to the specific needs in differing contexts. Médecins Sans Frontières (MSF), for example, offers opportunities for a range of qualified child health professionals to work principally in contexts affected by conflict, natural disasters and epidemic diseases. The Royal College of Paediatrics and Child Health (RCPCH) runs the Global Links programme, which facilitates placements of UK paediatricians in contexts most appropriate to their training and subspecialty interests, as well as the needs of the host institution. Reciprocally, the RCPCH Global Links programme also organizes placements in the UK for paediatricians from low-resource settings who have a particular subspecialty interest they wish to pursue. Some examples of getting involved are outlined in the following case study.

Case study

Peter is a paediatrician in training who has wanted to work in sub-Saharan Africa since his medical student elective in Malawi. He is keen on working in a district-level hospital in an area with a high prevalence of HIV and TB. After his third year of UK training, he applied to work with the Volunteer Service Overseas (VSO) organization, under a joint fellowship with his postgraduate college, the RCPCH. In preparation for his application, he attended various courses and meetings in global child health and gained teaching experience as an accredited Advanced Paediatric Life Support instructor. His application was successful and he gained unparalleled experience in tropical paediatrics in a Kenyan regional-level hospital for one year. He remained involved in global child health activities on his return to the UK, including advocacy work with UNICEF.

Charlotte was an experienced nurse working in the paediatric emergency department of a children's hospital in Quebec. She enjoyed working with the local African immigrant communities and had always wanted to spend time working in a low-resource setting for humanitarian reasons. She applied to Operation Smile, an NGO running programmes for cleft lip/palate repair in low-resource settings where there would otherwise be no access to treatment for this birth defect. Charlotte was successful in making it through the recruitment process – her clinical experience and her ability to speak French were particularly valuable. She enjoyed her first two-week mission to the Democratic Republic of Congo. Her husband was supportive and helped look after their two school-age children while she was away. Afterwards, she went on similar short missions annually and became a medical adviser to the Operation Smile office in Quebec.

CONCLUSION

Although there has been remarkable progress in reducing child mortality rates globally, the MDG 4 target will not be achieved in many countries. Much better information on mortality rates, health status and the effectiveness and coverage of interventions has allowed a better roll-out of community health programmes, but much work is still needed. The problem lies less with knowing which interventions work and more with ensuring that those interventions we know work effectively reach those most in need.

Although improved disease prevention and management are undoubtedly important, the greatest influences on child health are not medical. Economic status and maternal education remain the most protective factors for any child. As well as excellent clinical management of individual children, those working in child health in low-resource settings must also be effective advocates of education, especially of girls, and against child poverty.

REFERENCES

Bhutta, Z., Das, J.K., Walker, N., Rizvi, A., Campbell, H., Ruda, I., Black, R.E. (2013) 'Interventions to address deaths from childhood pneumonia and diarrhoea equitably: what works and at what cost?', *The Lancet*, 381(9875): 1417–1429.

Darmstadt, G.L., Bhutta, Z.A., Cousens, S., Adam, T., Walker, N., de Bernis, L. et al. (2005) 'Evidence-based, cost-effective interventions: how many newborn babies can we save?', *The Lancet*, 365(9463): 977–988.

Dondorp, A.M., Fanello, C.I., Hendriksen, I.C., Gomes, E., Seni, A., Chhaganlal, K.D. et al. (2010) 'Artesunate versus quinine in the treatment of severe falciparum malaria in African children (AQUAMAT): an open-label, randomised trial', *The Lancet*, 376(9753): 1647–1657.

Jackson, C., Mann, A., Mangtani, P.et al. (2012) 'Systematic review of observational data on effectiveness of *Haemophilus influenzae* type b (Hib) vaccines to allow optimization of vaccination schedules'. Available at: www.who.int/immunization/sage/meetings/2012/november/4._Systematic_review_of_observational_data_on_effectiveness_of_Hib_vaccines_Jackson_C_et_al_2012.pdf (accessed 8 October 2015).

Li Liu, L., Oza, S., Hogan, D., Perin, J., Rudan, I., Lawn, J.E., Cousens, S., Mathers, C. and Black, R.E. (2015) 'Global, regional, and national causes of child mortality in 2000–13, with projections to inform post-2015 priorities: an updated systematic analysis', *The Lancet*, 385: 430–440.

Luby, S.P., Agboatwalla, M., Feikin, D.R., Painter, J., Billhimer, W., Altaf, A. et al. (2005) 'Effect of handwashing on child health: a randomised controlled trial', *The Lancet*, 366(9481): 225–233.

Maitland, K., Kiguli, S., Opoka, R.O., Engoru, C., Olupot-Olupot, P., Akech, S.O. et al. (2011) 'Mortality after fluid bolus in African children with severe infection', *N Engl J Med*, 364(26): 2483–2495.

Martines, J., Paul, V.K., Bhutta, Z.A., Koblinsky, M., Soucat, A., Walker, N. et al. (2005) 'Neonatal survival: a call for action', *The Lancet*, 365(9465): 1189–1197.

Nelson, G.S. (1986) 'Hydatid disease: research and control in Turkana, Kenya. 1. Epidemiological observations', *Trans Royal Soc. Trop. Med, & Hygiene*, 80(2): 177–182.

UNICEF (2013) *Committing to Child Survival: A Promise Renewed. Progress Report.* Available at: www.childinfo.org/files/Child_Mortality_Report_2013.pdf (accessed 16 September 2013).

Violari, A., Cotton, M.F., Gibb, D.M., Babiker, A.G., Steyn, J., Madhi, S.A. et al.(2008) 'Early antiretroviral therapy and mortality among HIV-infected infants', *N Engl J Med.*, 359(21): 2233–2244.

Walker, C. L. F., Rudan, I., Liu, L., Nair, H., Theodoratou, E., Bhutta, Z. A. et al. (2013) 'Global burden of childhood pneumonia and diarrhoea', *The Lancet*, 381(9875), 1405–1416.

WHO (2008) *World Report on Injury Prevention*. Geneva: World Health Organization.

14

GLOBAL SURGERY

CHRIS LAVY, NYENGO MKANDAWIRE AND GODFREY MUGUTI

Chapter overview

After reading this chapter you will be able to:

- define 'global surgery'
- describe the differences between surgery in HICs and LICs
- explain measures to reduce the disparities in the availability of surgical services globally
- explain what can be done to make surgery sustainable.

INTRODUCTION

This chapter examines three aspects of surgery that have a global perspective. First, we outline the disparities that exist across the world in terms of surgical conditions and the management that is available for them. Second, we consider ways in which the disparities can be reduced and the gaps in surgical care bridged. Third, we look at some ways in which improvements in global surgery can be made sustainable. Inevitably, a short chapter like this will have to be selective in what it covers. Our experience has been mainly in Africa, so our illustrations will mainly be taken from that continent. The lessons learned and the important issues apply universally, however.

DISPARITIES IN GLOBAL SURGERY

Disparities exist in the types and volumes of pathology and their severity, as well as in available resources, including staff.

TYPES AND VOLUMES OF PATHOLOGY

Certain pathologies are much more common in some areas of the world than others and these disparities in prevalence inevitably affect the types of surgery needed. Sigmoid volvulus, for example, is rare in Western Europe and the USA, but, in the Peruvian Andes and sub-Saharan Africa, it causes up to 80 per cent of reported cases of intestinal obstruction (Asbun et al., 1992). Many infective conditions have a prevalence that varies widely across the world. Trachoma, an infection of the conjunctiva by the chlamydia organism, which can cause scarring of the eyelids and eventual blindness, is much more common in tropical countries than in temperate zones. Bacterial meningitis is also more common in tropical countries, leading to post-infective or obstructive hydrocephalus, which has a much higher prevalence in Uganda (Warf and Warf, 2010) than in the UK.

Every year, 5.8 million people die from musculoskeletal trauma and other injuries. These deaths are not evenly distributed, however, as 95 per cent of them occur in LMICs. This accounts for 10 per cent of the world's deaths – 32 per cent more than the fatalities from HIV/AIDS, TB and malaria combined. For every person who dies from trauma, approximately six times as many are injured, with temporary or permanent disabilities as a result. The appropriate management of this trauma requires surgical skills and facilities.

What is the evidence?

- About 1.24 million people die each year as a result of road traffic accidents.
- Road traffic injuries are the leading cause of death among young people, aged 15 to 29 years.
- Some 91 per cent of the world's fatalities on the roads occur in LMICs, even though these countries have approximately half of the world's vehicles.

Source: Data from the WHO (at: www.who.int/mediacentre/factsheets/fs358).

SEVERITY OF PATHOLOGY

Untreated common surgical conditions often deteriorate, moving from being mild to severe and even untreatable. Untreated inguinal hernias in Africa have been known to extend as far as the knee and contain most of the large bowel, requiring complex surgery to effect a repair. Similarly, club foot that is not treated early also deteriorates and may become irreducible without major surgery. Such conditions are examples of the kinds of deterioration in pathology that can occur when early treatment is not available and this forms part of the argument for making basic global surgical services available and, of course, awareness of, and early referral to, these services.

RESOURCES

Many of the disparities in surgical services on a global level are linked to funding. The WHO ranks countries according to how much is spent on healthcare on a per capita basis. In 2008, this varied from $10 per person per year in Eritrea and $12 in Myanmar (now Burma) to $3771 in the UK and $8019 in Norway. It is clear that there is a direct link between the amount of money spent and the availability of surgical equipment and consumables. Later in this chapter you'll see how this is also linked to surgical activity.

STAFFING DISPARITY

An enormous global disparity exists in the distribution of health workers of all types globally. For example, sub-Saharan Africa has 25 per cent of the global disease burden, yet only 3 per cent of the global health workers.

Activity 14.1

Visit the Worldmapper website (at: www.worldmapper.org) and find the map that displays the relative surface area of countries according to how many doctors they have working there. Note down what you learn from this map.

Comment

I'm sure you were not surprised by the inflated size of the USA and Canada and Europe. Africa looks like a burst balloon in comparison and Australia fares little better. Remember, this shows the numbers of all types of doctors, which may include traditional medical practitioners in East Asia.

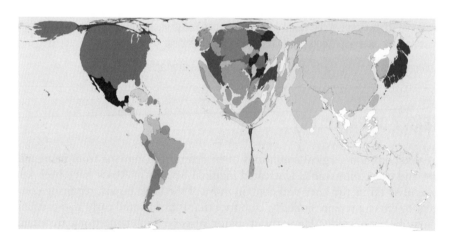

Figure 14.1   Distribution of doctors worldwide

Source: With permission of Worldmapper

The Royal College of Surgeons of England estimates that there are approximately 150 consultant surgeons (in all specialties) per million of the population in England and Wales. The College of Surgeons of East, Central and Southern Africa, in its most recent survey in 2011, estimates that the equivalent figure for Zambia and Zimbabwe is six per million, while for Malawi and Ethiopia the situation is slightly worse, with only four per million, which is 3 per cent of the UK figure.

DISPARITIES IN ACTIVITY

Inevitably, massive disparities in health funding and surgical staff result in fewer operations being performed. Weiser et al. (2008) mapped surgical activity on a global level and showed that the richest third of the world's population underwent 73.6 per cent of the world's surgical operations, while the poorest third underwent 3.5 per cent. They estimated that the richest countries have a surgical operation rate per 100,000 of the population which is 100 times that of the poorest countries, plus there is an almost perfect correlation between the logarithms of per capita expenditure on health and the amount of surgery performed.

What is the evidence?

What types of surgery are carried out in district hospitals in LICs?

We did a survey of the surgical activities of all the district hospitals in Malawi over a one-year period in 2003 (Lavy et al., 2007). The results (see Figure 14.2) showed that dilatation and curettage (D&C) was the most common type of operation, closely followed by caesarian section. Other types of surgery, including laparotomy, were much less common. We concluded that a caesarian section was a relatively straightforward operation and, in an emergency situation, could not be referred elsewhere so had to be performed at the district level. Other operations did not have such a degree of urgency and so could be referred to bigger hospitals.

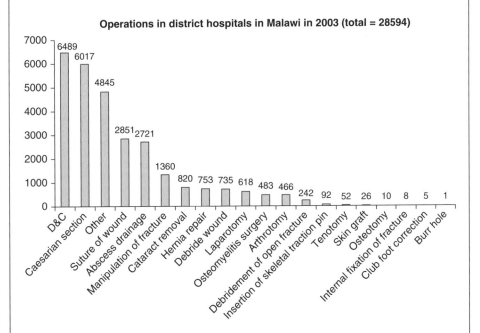

Figure 14.2   Types of surgery carried out in district hospitals in Malawi in 2003

Source: Lavy et al. (2007)

BRIDGING THE GAPS IN GLOBAL SURGERY

This section looks at some initiatives to address the disparities we have noted, such as training, task shifting and concentrating on provision in district hospitals. Short-term visits from overseas professionals also contribute.

TRAINING

It is impossible in a chapter to cover the topic of surgical training at a global level and there are many excellent university-based training schemes around the world, so we will, instead simply highlight three initiatives aimed at increasing the number of surgeons and, thus, surgical capacity.

The College of Surgeons of East, Central and Southern Africa (COSECSA) represents a region of the world where there are very few surgeons. It has therefore put together a training scheme that will add to the existing university postgraduate training programmes in the region and increase the number of trainee places for surgery.

COSECSA has reviewed all the hospitals in its region and selected those where there are good standards to host trainees. It has a rigorous system of assessment to monitor trainee surgeons and an annual examination diet to allow these trainees to progress through the five-year postgraduate courses that lead to the COSECSA fellowship and the ability to practice surgery as a specialist in the region. The fact that COSECSA's training is all local mitigates the brain drain that is more likely when surgeons train abroad, plus the breadth of its courses, spanning most surgical specialties, encourages graduates to choose a local career path and professional development.

The Pan African Association of Christian Surgeons (PAACS) has done a similar thing in both West and East Africa. It has identified well-run mission hospitals where there is capacity for training and takes on candidates who follow a five-year structured training programme, leading to a certificate in surgical competence given by a leading American university.

The West African College of Surgeons (WACS) predates COSECSA and was one of the models on which COSECSA is based. WACS includes both francophone and anglophone countries and offers its exams in both languages and its annual congresses include bilingual presentations.

TASK SHIFTING

It is clear that there is an enormous burden of disease at a global level that needs surgical treatment, but, in many countries, insufficient surgeons are available to meet that need. Training more surgeons is part of the solution. Not all surgical procedures need to be performed by postgraduate surgeons, however – clinicians with a reduced level of training can perform at least some of them.

Such reassignment of duties to other cadres has been termed 'task shifting' by the WHO. There have been several very successful task-shifting programmes in resource-poor settings. In Mozambique, a group of clinicians named 'technicos' have been trained to perform a number of basic surgical procedures, including caesarian sections, and a review of their results shows that their success rate, including infection rates, are similar to those achieved by medically qualified surgeons (Vaz et al., 1999).

In Malawi, a programme of training non-medically qualified clinicians in orthopaedic and trauma treatment was started in 1985 (Mkandawire et al., 2008). These orthopaedic clinical officers are able to treat more than 80 per cent of the trauma and injury cases that present at district hospitals in Malawi and, in many ways, are a more appropriate level of clinician to have offering this treatment at these rural hospitals. As well as their clinical skills at treating injuries, the orthopaedic clinical officers in Malawi have been shown to have a level of success in the manipulation and casting of club feet that is indistinguishable from that of fully trained physiotherapists and orthopaedic surgeons (Tindall et al., 2005).

Task shifting has many benefits where the population is large and the number of surgeons is small. It is therefore of prime importance that clinical officers or technicos and surgeons work closely together, teaching each other, learning from each other's experiences and sharing the surgical workload. It must be said, however, that as the number of surgeons increases, then the division of labour may have to be reviewed. In Malawi and Zambia there are now established career paths for non-physician clinicians at a BSc university level. COSTAFRICA is a combined Royal College of Surgeons in Ireland/European Union training and research programme that is evaluating the training and work of these essential surgical practitioners.

Activity 14.2

If you were in charge of surgery in a country of one million people and had two surgeons and ten non-medically qualified clinicians, how would you organize the surgical services?

Comment

Mkandawire et al.'s (2008: 2391) paper recommends that, 'orthopaedic surgeons are trained to provide specialist services at central and referral hospitals and also assist in training and mentoring orthopaedic clinical officers. Orthopaedic services must be brought nearer to the population by training more orthopaedic clinical officers and deploying them in rural, district, and mission hospitals where the majority of the population lives. Each such hospital must have at least one orthopaedic clinician.'

CONCENTRATING ON PROVISION IN DISTRICT HOSPITALS

The above two sections have concentrated on increasing the numbers of both surgeons and non-medically qualified personnel who can perform surgery. This section looks at where they work.

There is a tendency for people in LMICs gaining additional educational skills and qualifications to move to urban areas. This is natural as it is often in such areas that they are trained and where medical facilities are often better resourced. There is a good side to this, as urban areas are more densely populated and have their own surgical needs, which increase as the urban areas grow. There is, however, a tendency for the rural areas to become relatively depleted of healthcare workers and, especially, of surgeons. If market forces are left to guide where a country's surgical resources are located, then they will tend to accumulate in towns and big cities, where they can serve those who can afford to pay the surgeons.

Ignoring market economic forces is unrealistic, but there is great wisdom in improving rural health services. The district hospital is usually the lowest level of health institution that has a functioning operating theatre and, if these theatres can be maintained, then surgical treatment can be offered to a large number of rural and peri-urban people. Several countries have, therefore, encouraged medical staff to move to rural district hospitals by making life more attractive there. These attractions may take the form of cheaper housing or enhanced pay.

Maintaining a functioning operating theatre in a district hospital provides both a location where general surgical emergencies and trauma can be treated and a place where obstetric emergencies can be dealt with. A theatre that is well equipped for general and trauma surgery is also one that is ready and available for caesarian sections. The authors and colleagues have found that theatres where safe caesarian sections are performed are also able to host many other types of surgery.

Several other authors have also observed that the number of caesarian sections performed is a relatively good proxy measure for the availability of surgical facilities in a region (Reshamwalla et al., 2012). Caesarian sections are a common, relatively simple emergency operation and, where facilities and expertise allow, they are usually carried out.

The WHO estimates that approximately 10 per cent of pregnancies require a caesarian section or some kind of operative intervention. Some HICs have a caesarian section rate of almost 25 per cent, but it is likely that issues other than urgent medical need have some bearing on this. At the other end of the spectrum, in countries where the caesarian section rate is below 10 per cent, the reason is usually that surgical facilities or expertise are in short supply. In parts of Malawi, Ethiopia and Niger, the rate is around 2 to 3 per cent (Betrán et al., 2007). This means that many mothers and unborn babies suffer prolonged and potentially harmful deliveries or death. It also means that if caesarian sections cannot be performed safely, then general surgical services are unlikely to be as they use the very same facilities.

SHORT-TERM SURGICAL TRIPS FROM RICHER COUNTRIES

Possibly many readers of this book will have been on a short-term trip to a resource-poor country; indeed their interest in global health may have been stimulated by such a visit. There are many good aspects to such trips, in that patients who need surgery often receive it, some local surgeons receive a degree of training and the visitors from richer countries develop a deeper understanding of global issues, the disparity of resources on our planet and, often, a deeper appreciation of their own health systems. The NHS, for example, might seem wonderful after returning from a country with minimal health services.

Potentially bad, unhelpful and unintended consequences of such short-term trips should also always be considered before they are arranged. For example, these trips can raise the expectations of local people to such a degree that they wait for the next visiting surgeon rather than seeing and being treated by a local surgeon. The overall effect is thus one of discouragement for the local health service. We have heard of trips where the queue of excited people coming to see the visiting team was so big that there was suffocation and death in the crowd.

Equally, the members of the visiting team may be more interested in seeing rare and interesting cases and training other members of their own team than in building local capacity and training local surgeons.

The trip may also have been organized with no reference to local clinicians. We have experienced this when Church-related organizations have arranged clinics in rural areas. Visiting surgeons who don't know the local facilities may well take on cases that are too complex for the local theatre and recovery team. We have seen death and paralysis occur when surgery by well-meaning visitors has been too ambitious. Also, surgical trips may leave complications that occur after the visiting team has gone and the host team is not sure quite what to do.

Case study

A visiting spinal surgeon from the USA had operated on hundreds of cases of scoliosis (curvature of the spine) in New York, with excellent results. He visited a small African country with a complete theatre team and operated on a teenage boy with a severe curve. He was not used to the theatre facilities and he did not have the spinal cord monitoring equipment that he was used to. The operation went well and the spine was perfectly straight. When the boy came round from the anaesthetic, however, he was paralysed from the waist down.

- Should the surgeon have performed the operation without his spinal cord monitoring equipment?
- Should the surgeon have accepted a partial correction that was less good cosmetically but also less likely to stretch the spinal cord?
- Should the surgeon have done the operation at all if this kind of surgery was not routinely done in that country?

We do not want to be negative about well-meaning attempts to help by surgeons from richer countries, but such trips should be well organized and link in with existing healthcare and training facilities. The impetus and the direction should be local and the whole trip should empower, enhance and develop local capacity through sustainable partnerships and collaborations.

Activity 14.3

If you were asked by a disability charity in a LIC to organize a team of plastic surgeons to come out and operate on the many cases of cleft lip and palate in a certain location, how would you do it?

(Continued)

(Continued)

- Who would you contact for information?
- Would you seek permission? If so, from whom?
- Who would you bring and why?
- Who would you try to work with?
- Are there any situations into which you would feel it best not to go?

Comment

Two publications are helpful here. The first is by Grimes et al. (2013), which outlines the criteria for setting up a successful visiting surgical project. The second is a booklet by the Christian Medical Fellowship on short-term medical visits (Lavy, 2013). It is mainly based on the experiences gained from mission-linked visits, but the lessons learned are valuable for all.

MAKING GLOBAL SURGERY SUSTAINABLE

In this last section, we look at ways of trying to make surgical delivery more sustainable in resource-poor settings. We will start by saying that this is hard! It is hard in the UK to stop health costs spiralling out of control and that is in a country where an annual sum of approximately £2500 ($3771) is spent per person per year on health. How hopeful can we be, then, that sustainability is possible in countries such as Eritrea where the people are poor and the annual per capita expenditure on health is £8, which is 0.3 per cent of the UK's?

DISPEL MISCONCEPTIONS

It has often been thought that surgery is the expensive icing on the cake of a health system. That, when trying to improve the health of a population, one starts with preventive measures, such as ensuring there is clean water and good nutrition, then moves to other cheap, effective things, such as vaccinations, then to medical treatment, which involves drugs and antibiotics, and only when all these other things have been sorted out should a country start to be involved in the expense of surgery, with its massive unit costs per patient.

We feel this is a myth that should be dispelled. When one does the calculations, the cost of surgery in terms of DALYs averted, it compares very favourably with the treatment of other conditions (Figure 14.3).

What is the evidence?

Is surgery cost-effective?

DALY measurement is a technique used by the WHO to look at the cost-effectiveness of a treatment. It is assumed, purely for the sake of calculation, that a year of a life lived with an illness or curable condition is of less value than one lived without that condition and, for the purposes of calculation, the illness or condition is given an estimated weighting or percentage by which it reduces the value or quality of that one year of life. If a treatment can cure or help that illness for the rest of the patient's life, then a calculation can be done on how many remaining years of life are improved – or DALYs averted – for the cost of that cure. Thus, treatments can be compared according to the cost of averting one DALY.

This is a methodology that has limitations and critics, but it is used as a standard in health economics and it is generally agreed that treatments averting a DALY for less than $100 are good value.

It had been assumed that DALYs averted by surgery would be expensive, but a number of recently published papers show that surgery is very cost-effective compared to common standard treatments that are administered as part of public health measures, as shown in Table 14.1.

Table 14.1   Cost-effectiveness of interventions

Surgical interventions	Cost in US$ per DALY averted
Hernia repair	12–78
Emergency caesarian section	18+
Cleft lip repair	15–96
Trauma surgery	32–233
Non-surgical interventions	
Oral rehydration	1062
Vitamin A supplementation	6–12
Breastfeeding promotion	930
ART for HIV	922

Source: Grimes et al. (2014)

Another misconception about surgery is the belief that internal fixation and the use of surgical implants in HIV-positive patients should be avoided as the likelihood of infection is inevitable. This has resulted in many HIV-positive patients being denied appropriate surgery, but careful research has shown the myth to be unfounded (Harrison et al., 2002).

STIMULATE GLOBAL INTEREST AND RESEARCH

The work on DALYs mentioned in the previous section has only taken place because of the recent increase in interest in global surgical research. Surgeons have always been interested and involved in clinical work in resource-poor areas of the world, but the physical excitement and technical challenge of the work has often been so great that it has left little time for research. A literature review of surgery in Africa showed that very little surgical research comes out of resource-poor countries (Lavy et al., 2011).

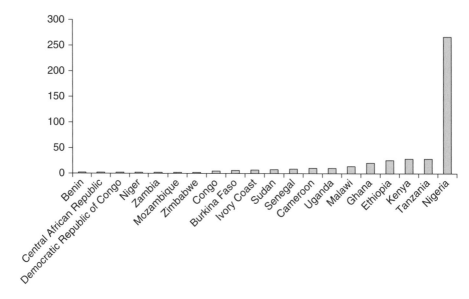

Figure 14.3   The total scientific papers in all surgical disciplines in Africa published in one year

Source: Lavy et al. (2011)

The last decade has shown a major increase in interest in global surgery as a topic for research elsewhere, however. Easy travel, the Internet, access to knowledge about the major disparities in global surgery and the realization that there are many poorly understood surgical conditions, are all reasons for global surgical research becoming an increasingly popular area of study. Many surgeons in both rich and poor countries are reawakening to the reason they first went into medicine: to make a difference. This is to be welcomed and there have been various organizations set up to stimulate and encourage surgery, research and teaching in resource-poor settings. Some of these are listed at the end of this chapter.

The new research agenda for global surgery should concentrate on the problems of LICs and focus on the burden of disease, surgical outcomes, safe surgery and increasing their capacity to treat people. It is our hope that there will be a reversal of the current 90/10 bottleneck – that is, 90 per cent of research funds allocated globally support the surgical problems of the most affluent 10 per cent of the world's population.

INTERNATIONAL COOPERATION ON WORKFORCE PLANNING

The brain drain of skills and manpower from LICs to HICs is not new, nor simple. There are many reasons and factors involved in healthcare professionals relocating to other counties. The economics of such moves is also very complicated and sometimes the donor country benefits economically when a doctor moves from a poorer to a richer region and sends a large proportion of the salary home. Some countries, such as the Philippines, produce and train far more health professionals than they need specifically to export them and benefit from what they send home and return with. This model could well be looked at by other LICs. Exporting skills in this way is possibly more economically effective in the long term than exporting raw materials.

From a global perspective, it is encouraging to see the formation of groups of surgeons in the diaspora (the community that has left a country to go to another place) meeting together to look at how they can be involved in improving surgery in the countries where they were born. It is also encouraging to see the formation, in the UK, of the Zambia– and the Uganda–UK Healthcare Workforce Alliances Although not specifically surgical, they promote the networking of UK-based organizations that are associated with healthcare work in the linked country with the ministries of health in those countries, with the aim of improving the size, training and efficiency of the healthcare workforce in Uganda and Zambia.

FUNDING MODELS

Surgery falls into two categories of funding model. Elective procedures, such as joint replacement, hernia, skin lesions and prostate problems are actively sought out by the rich and influential in any society. If these conditions in this section of the population are not catered for appropriately in the patients' own countries, then they will travel overseas to have their problem fixed, with all the implications of loss of income to the home countries, as it is spent instead in the countries they travel to, and failure to promote local services that involves.

Surgical conditions affecting poorer people that are not life-threatening and unlikely to be priorities for LMICs include severe club foot and angular limb deformity.

If, however, the richer and the poorer groups can be brought together, then there can be symbiosis. The first group's fees can help equip and fund a unit that the second group can benefit from, too. We have never yet met rich patients who are not happy to hear that their reasonable fees helped build capacity in their country and fund surgery for others less fortunate than them.

This funding model is not in any way the panacea for LMICs health problems, but change is often not made in massive jumps but incrementally and this is one such small, but purposeful jump that surgery can take in the right direction.

SURGEONS AS ADVOCATES

The best spokespeople for the job of improving global understanding and support for surgery are probably surgeons themselves. Compared with other groups of clinicians in the past, surgeons have not been interested in global statistics, global campaigns and public health issues. It is now time for this to change.

Surgery, and the people who suffer from surgical conditions, deserve representation at the top table in global health discussions at the WHO and it is the duty of surgeons to be advocates.

Activity 14.4

If you were asked to help with the surgical section of the five-year health services plan for a low-income country, what would be the key items you would suggest?

Comment

You might like to refer back to the 'What is the evidence?' box earlier in this chapter. The use of DALYs as a measure of value for money means clashes between different components of healthcare can be resolved equitably.

EMPOWERING MINISTRIES OF HEALTH

Nigel Crisp's book *Turning the World Upside Down* (2010), talks of a meeting with the Minister of Health in Mozambique who said that he was really the Minister for health projects that were run by foreigners. There is indeed a tendency for many well-meaning foreign organizations to come to LMICs, set up offices and then work hard within their own boundaries to improve healthcare. While this dream is laudable, it is not always practical, nor sustainable and it is often pursued without any reference to national health plans.

Ministries of health are not always efficient, nor, indeed, free of internal issues, both financial and organizational, but the fact remains that each is responsible for its country and its healthcare, including its surgical healthcare. Any foreign assistance or health project in a country absolutely has to fit in with the healthcare planning for that country and play its part in empowering and building up the ministry of health and its offices.

It is possible, in the short term, to run a project that delivers surgical services to a LMIC using external funds in isolation from its national health services. In the long term, however, the best way forward is to acknowledge the leadership of the ministry of health, work in close, open and transparent collaboration with them and use any resources that come in to build up individuals and capacity in that ministry of health. Ministries of health are not perfect, but they are responsible for change and improvement. NGOs may be well organized, but they may not be there in ten years. The ministries of health will.

CONCLUSION

Huge disparities exist throughout the world concerning people's access to surgery that are not based on clinical need, but, primarily, on economic and social grounds. This results in some groups not having access to surgery for what might be considered minor or routine conditions in HICs, as many LMICs struggle to provide adequate surgical services.

The cost of this lack of access to surgery is very high, in terms of both mortality and morbidity. A range of initiatives exist to help address this shortfall, ranging from international and national policy initiatives, international partnerships and collaborations, task shifting and training.

ORGANIZATIONS AND USEFUL WEBSITES

Alliance for Surgery and Anesthesia Presence (ASAP): http://asaptoday.org

Global Alliance for Surgery, Obstetrics, Trauma and Anesthesia Care (G4 Alliance): www.theg4alliance.org

Global Partners in Anaesthesia and Surgery: www.globalpas.org

Institute for Global Orthopaedics and Traumatology: http://orthosurg.ucsf.edu

International Collaboration for Essential Surgery: http://essentialsurgery.com

International Development Committee: www.internationalsurgery.org.uk

The Lancet Commission on Global Surgery: www.thelancet.com/commissions/global-surgery

World Orthopaedic Concern UK: www.wocuk.org

WHO Global Initiative for Emergency and Essential Surgical Care: www.who.int/surgery/globalinitiative

REFERENCES

Asbun, H., Castellanos, H., Balderrama, B., Ochoa, J., Arismendi, R., Teran, H., et al. (1992) 'Sigmoid volvulus in the high altitude of the Andes. Review of 230 cases', *Dis Colon Rectum*, 35(4): 350–353.

Betrán, A., Merialdi, M., Lauer, J., Bing-Shun, W., Thomas, J., Van Look, P., et al. (2007) 'Rates of caesarean section: analysis of global, regional and national estimates', *Paediatr Perinat Epidemiol*, 21(2): 98–113.

Crisp, N. (2010) *Turning the World Upside Down*. Boca Raton, Florida: CRC Press.

Grimes, C.E., Henry, J.A., Maraka, J., Mkandawire, N.C. and Cotton, M. (2014) 'Cost-effectiveness of surgery in low and middle-income countries: a systematic review', *World J Surg*, 38(1): 252–263.

Grimes, C.E., Maraka, J., Kingsnorth, A.N., Darko, R., Samkange, C.A. and Lane, R.H. (2013) 'Guidelines for surgeons on establishing projects in low-income countries', *World J Surg*, 37(6): 1203–1207.

Harrison, W.J., Lewis, C.P. and Lavy, C.B. (2002) 'Wound healing after implant surgery in HIV-positive patients', *J Bone Joint Surg Br*, 84(6): 802–806.

Lavy, C., Tindall, A., Steinlechner, C., Mkandawire, N. and Chimangemi, S. (2007) 'Surgery in Malawi: a national survey of activity in rural and urban hospitals', *Ann R Coll Surg Engl*, 89(7): 722–724.

Lavy, C., Sauven, K., Mkandawire, N., Charian, M., Gosselin, R., Ndihokubwayo, J.B., et al. (2011) 'State of surgery in tropical Africa: a review', *World J Surg*, 35(2): 262–271.

Lavy, V. (2013) *Short Term Medical Work. CMF ISBN* 9780906747490.

Mkandawire, N.C., Ngulube, C. and Lavy, C. (2008) 'Orthopaedic clinical officer program in Malawi: a model for providing orthopaedic care', *Clin Orthop Relat Res,* 466(10): 2385–2391.

Reshamwalla, S., Gobeze, A., Ghosh, S., Grimes, C. and Lavy, C. (2012) 'Snapshot of surgical activity in rural Ethiopia: is enough being done?', *World J Surg,* 36(5): 1049–1055.

Tindall, A.J., Steinlechner, C.W., Lavy, C.B., Mannion, S. and Mkandawire, N. (2005) 'Results of manipulation of idiopathic clubfoot deformity in Malawi by orthopaedic clinical officers using the Ponseti method: a realistic alternative for the developing world?', *J Pediatr Orthop,* 25(5): 627–629.

Vaz, F., Bergström, S., Vaz Mda, L., Langa, J. and Bugalho, A. (1999) 'Training medical assistants for surgery', *Bull World Health Org,* 77(8): 688–691.

Warf, B. and Warf, C. (2010) 'Pediatric hydrocephalus in East Africa: prevalence, causes, treatments, and strategies for the future', *World Neurosurg,* 73(4): 296–300.

Weiser, T., Regenbogen, S., Thompson, K., Haynes, A.B., Lipsitz, S.R., Berry, W.R., et al. (2008) 'An estimation of the global volume of surgery: a modelling strategy based on available data', *The Lancet,* 372(9633): 139–144.

15

GLOBAL EMERGENCY CARE AND DISASTER HEALTH

GEORGINA PHILLIPS, AMY NEILSON AND ROB MITCHELL

Chapter overview

After reading this chapter you will be able to:

- describe global emergency care (GEC) as a multidisciplinary, horizontally based practice, and its role in functional health systems
- show how practitioners can improve patient outcomes through GEC work
- explain the epidemiology of disasters in relation to underlying health systems
- appreciate the importance of professionalism and accountability in disaster response
- define the skills, knowledge and attributes required for safe and effective GEC practice
- describe the options for professionals to gain experience early in their careers in the delivery of emergency care in low-resource environments.

INTRODUCTION

DEFINITIONS AND SCOPE

Emergency care (EC) encompasses clinical service provision, capacity development and health systems strengthening to handle acute and urgent aspects of illness and injury.

Global emergency care (GEC) emphasizes the transnational aspects of disease and healthcare, the synthesis of public health and clinical care and the pursuit of equity across populations.

The International Federation for Emergency Medicine (IFEM) has defined the breadth of emergency medicine (EM) practice: it is for all injuries, all illnesses and all ages; it involves prevention as well as management and it includes systems of care both outside and inside the hospital. This equally well describes GEC; a more inclusive term that acknowledges the team-based and multidisciplinary practice of EC, which can also occur in hospitals as well as community and rural health clinics.

As a horizontal discipline, EC works across vertical silos of care in an integrative way. Being population-based, it reflects the demographics and health problems of the whole community. GEC includes development activities (building capacity in emergency care systems), as well as disaster health and humanitarian assistance. The relationship between these interrelated disciplines is shown in Figure 15.1. Disaster health, an important field in its own right, is considered in the second section of this chapter. A detailed discussion of humanitarian action, including the response to complex emergencies, is, however, beyond the scope of this chapter.

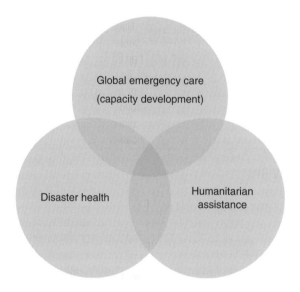

Figure 15.1 Global emergency care and related disciplines

EC IN LMICS

This section considers the 'What?' and 'Why?' of EC.

-- Activity 15.1 --

You are on medical placement to a provincial hospital in Papua New Guinea. During your shift in the busy 'emergency/outpatients' section, a nurse brings in a mother with her drowsy five-year-old daughter, who is struggling to breathe. They had been waiting in the queue to see the doctor for three hours, but now her condition has worsened. With the help of other staff, you attempt to resuscitate the child, but the room is crowded, poorly equipped and very hot. She needs fluids (but IV access is difficult), oxygen, some breathing support and a focused assessment to work out what the diagnosis is.

In time, it emerges that she was bitten on her bare foot by a snake last night while playing in long grass. There was no first aid given.

Later in the day, you also see four very dehydrated people from the same village with watery diarrhoea and manage a young man with head, chest and abdominal injuries from a motorbike accident.

List all of the components of EC that you had to deal with today. What made the outcomes for your patients potentially worse? What helped?

Comment

This is a typical day in any emergency department, resource-rich or poor. Urgent health needs encompass the broad spectrum of illness and injury. For the child with a snakebite, not only do you require good clinical skills in terms of assessment and resuscitation but also teamwork, collaboration with other disciplines (paediatrics) and to follow up outstanding issues (public health education and first aid training).

If there had been a functional triage system, the little girl's situation may have been identified earlier and not deteriorated while she was waiting. Having a well-designed and equipped acute treatment area makes an enormous difference to your ability to manage very unwell patients.

The four patients with diarrhoea may represent an infectious outbreak. The EC you are giving includes appropriate clinical care, infection control, liaison with inpatient units and following up such suspicions with public health and government authorities. Trauma care relies on having a skilled team and collaboration with many disciplines, such as surgery, lab, radiology and anaesthetics. You might be stimulated to start an audit on the type of trauma patients that are presenting to this hospital, or start a public health campaign on motorbike helmet safety.

GLOBAL DEVELOPMENT OF EM AND EC

EM emerged as a specialty discipline alongside improvements in emergency department (ED) function in North America, the UK and Australasia around 30–40 years ago (Curry, 2008). The most acute, unstable and undifferentiated patients require care by skilled clinicians working in appropriate environments.

Global recognition of EM as a medical specialty means the IFEM represents EM organizations across the world, from both LICs and HICs. It produces resources such as curriculum guidelines, quality and safety standards and a growing research base to support capacity development to improve EC.

Traditionally, global health and international aid and development workers have had a minimal understanding of how GEC fits in LMICs, believing it to pertain to healthcare in disaster situations only. Yet, more recent Global Burden of Disease data highlighted trauma and non-communicable diseases (NCDs) as major contributors to death and disease, currently under-addressed by the MDGs. In response, the post-2015 Sustainable Development Goals (SDGs) set specific targets for reducing mortality from road traffic accidents and NCDs, as well as focusing on substance abuse, mental health, equity of access to health services and improving the capacity of health systems and training of the health workforce. GEC activities have a crucial role to play in all of these areas, in addition to the ongoing work towards achieving the MDG targets.

People injured in accidents, new mothers with post-partum sepsis, dehydrated babies, suicidal young men and those with exacerbations of their chronic respiratory disease need to access safe and effective EC. A system meeting public expectations for accessible healthcare in urgent and life-threatening situations is necessary in any environment. Given the high and complex burden of disease in developing settings, the provision of safe and effective EC is even more important. Functional acute care systems not only improve the health of populations and meet public expectations but also facilitate effective responses in times of increased need (Razzak and Kellermann, 2002). The WHO advocates universal access to EC services.

THE IMPACT OF EFFECTIVE EC

The annual Global Emergency Medicine Literature Review reports new research in the field of EC in low-resource settings (Becker et al., 2014). Compelling evidence about the effectiveness of introducing a system of GEC comes from Malawi, through research that transformed a busy children's 'outpatients and emergency clinic' previously providing inadequate service with a high case–fatality rate (Molyneux et al., 2006). By training staff in emergency skills and knowledge, introducing systems of emergency care such as triage, better communication and improved patient flow, and redesigning the environment of care, improved functioning of the new 'emergency department' and a substantial reduction in patient mortality was demonstrated. This work has been pivotal in the development and global propagation of the simple and effective triage tool for children, Emergency Triage Assessment and Treatment (ETAT; WHO, 2005).

CHARACTERISTICS OF GEC ACTIVITIES

There are three core components to capacity development in GEC: staff skills and knowledge, EC systems and the environment in which EC is delivered. GEC activities may encompass any or all of these areas and often deliver clinical services and build capacity simultaneously. Furthermore, GEC activities are not confined to doctors. As GEC is a multidisciplinary, team-based practice, effective and sustainable GEC activities are best illustrated by programmes that incorporate medical, nursing, pre-hospital and administrative skills. Table 15.1 provides a framework for understanding the breadth of GEC service provision and activities that develop capacity, as illustrated by the Myanmar case study below.

Table 15.1　GEC activities

Category	Activity	
	Service provision	Capacity development
Staff skill and knowledge	• EC service provision in hospitals, clinics or the community • Disaster/crisis and complex emergency relief work	• Short training courses • Mentoring and peer support • Bedside and structured clinical teaching • Specialty-building programs; 　○ Medical 　○ Nursing 　○ Para-medical

Category	Activity	
	Service provision	**Capacity development**
		• Exchange visits between low-resource and mature system environments

GEC systems	• Pre-hospital systems
	  o Emergency Care delivery in pre-hospital or community settings
	• Triage
	  o Clinical emergency nursing work
	• Patient flow
	  o Clinical and administrative emergency work in hospitals or clinics
		o Work with local stakeholders to establish a pre-hospital system; (legislation, dispatch, vehicles, training programme, standards
		o ETAT short course training
		o Local triage tool development and implementation
		o Work with local staff to map patient traffic, reduce bottlenecks and delays in care

	• Communication o Clinical emergency work; modelling effective communication and collaboration across disciplines	o Clinical handover tool development o Interdisciplinary clinical guidelines and communication agreements
	• Patient information o Implementation of data management systems	o Hospital-wide training in data management systems and maintenance

	• Quality improvement
	  o Clinical EC work; evidence based and high quality
	  o Utilization of clinical protocols
		o Local clinical protocol development
		o Introduction of audits

Environment of care	• Emergency department design
	  o Renovation of EC space to improve function
	  o Creation of appropriate areas for resuscitation.
		o Development of emergency care design standards and guidelines

	• Equipment standards and implementation
	  o Provision of equipment for EC delivery
	  o Biomedical support for existing equipment
		o Development of minimum equipment requirements for EC
		o Sourcing of cost effective and repairable equipment

General	• Research
	  o Priorities include local burden of disease profile and outcome analysis of GEC system development and education activities
	• National standards
	  o Documentation of minimum local requirements for safe and effective emergency care
	• Integration and collaboration with policy and planning
	  o Advocacy for GEC into national health policy, budget and legislation	

Case study　The Myanmar EC programme

After Cyclone Nargis in 2008, the Myanmar Medical Association and Ministry of Health embarked on a comprehensive programme to improve EC for the country, beginning with a short course in trauma skills. Subsequently, an EM training programme for doctors, development of a pre-hospital ambulance system, rebuilding and renovating of hospital emergency departments and nurse training for EC were included. Partnership with the Australian Volunteers International organization allowed the long-term placement of emergency physicians, ambulance and nurse trainers, plus a network of clinicians from Hong Kong and Australia provided a substantial short-term volunteer workforce. Now, Myanmar doctors are leading the 'on the ground' teaching and training of local staff and advocating for EC improvements in their hospitals and clinics (Phillips et al., 2014).

DISASTER HEALTH

Disaster health delivers timely, skilled and appropriate additional resources as an adjunct to local health systems.

Disasters have traditionally been defined as natural or man-made and complex. These definitions are evolving. The term 'natural disaster' describes the effect of earthquakes, tropical cyclones, floods, tsunamis, droughts and other predominantly weather-related events on societies. Increasingly, these are becoming known as 'hazards', the effects of which may lead to a disaster. The phrase 'complex disasters' may be used to describe the adverse effects of conflict on populations.

This development is important because the traditional definitions fail to acknowledge that whether or not an event is a disaster depends less on the aetiology of the event than on the capacity of the society concerned to respond. Events such as the Ebola outbreak in West Africa throughout 2014 and beyond are neither natural, man-made, nor associated with war, yet strongly reflect underlying health and governance capability (see Chapter 3).

Complex humanitarian emergencies (CHE) are particularly challenging disasters. They are political, man-made occurrences, whereby events have led to marked human suffering, including but not limited to war, disease, hunger, inadequate housing, exposure to physical and psychological trauma and/or forced migration. CHEs are multidimensional and, predominantly, prolonged crises.

Responding to a potentially disastrous incident requires adequate EC systems, encompassing clinical service provision, capacity development and strengthening of health systems for all acute and urgent aspects of any illness and injury. Underlying systems and structures influence the capacity of a community to respond to an adverse incident. Poverty-stricken LMICs are particularly vulnerable to the effects of disasters, yet developed countries are not immune, as seen in the case of the 2011 earthquake in Christchurch, New Zealand.

In relation to four types of hazard – earthquake, tropical cyclone, flood and drought – countries classified at a high level of human development represent 15 per cent of the exposed population, but only 1.8 per cent of the deaths (UN, 2004). Development can both increase and decrease disaster risk. Rapid urbanization can put populations at increased risk of climate change and flood.

Activity 15.2

Search for and view meteorological images on the Internet, directly comparing Cyclone Yasi in 2011 and Hurricane Katrina in 2005. What else can you find out about these disasters?

Comment

Cyclone Yasi was 650 km wide, with winds up to 295 km an hour. Hurricane Katrina was 640 km wide, with winds up to 280 km an hour. Cyclone Yasi resulted in storm surges of up to five metres. It made landfall south of Innisfail, Queensland, Australia, devastating homes, commercial buildings, farms and livelihoods. One person is reported to have died as a result of Cyclone Yasi. Hurricane Katrina killed nearly 2000 people. Her storm surges ranged from 4.9 to 8.2 metres. The damage bill was estimated at US$91 billion.

These storms are comparable on a number of levels. Why did they have such differing impacts? Think about population density, overall population size, emergency preparedness and government responses prior and subsequent to the storm reaching landfall.

Disaster response is essentially a public health response to an exceptional incident. It may involve water and sanitation, provision of electricity, emergency housing, communications and other tasks, depending on the scenario. Health is one key aspect. Disaster health may require the scaling up of resources on the ground and the importation of variety of skilled professionals, depending on the nature of the incident and resultant devastation.

Activity 15.3

Consider the following health and related systems issues and rate them according to urgency.

- Trauma: physical effects.
- Trauma: psychological effects.
- Safe drinking water.
- Floods facilitating water-borne disease.
- Worsening of mosquito-borne disease.
- Victim search and rescue.

- Sourcing medications that need to be taken regularly (insulin, anti-convulsants and so on).
- Family reunification.
- Disabled people's needs.
- Safe burials.
- Safe shelter.
- Food and nutrition.

Did you find this difficult to do? Each of these may be equally important and require an equally timely response, hence the breadth of disciplines and contributors to disaster response and the importance of effective coordination.

Redmond (2005) describes three phases following the impact of an earthquake. The first three to seven days are focused on search and rescue and the management of acute trauma. The following weeks to months concentrate on surveillance of communicable diseases. Reconstruction and economic and social problems are then addressed over the ensuing months to years. Similar phases exist for the consequences of other hazards.

DEVELOPING DISASTER RESPONSE

Some of the roots of disaster healthcare lie in humanitarianism. The concept of the Red Cross began in 1839 as a response to the needs of wounded soldiers in Italy dying on the battlefield. The International Federation of Red Cross and Red Crescent Societies (IFRC) was formed in 1919 following World War I. Today, the International Red Cross and Red Crescent movement is the largest humanitarian network in the world, with 189 national societies across the globe. Among other activities, it coordinates and directs international assistance following natural and man-made disasters in non-conflict situations. In the setting of a disaster, national societies are already on the ground and constitute the key response. The IFRC augments this response when called on by the national societies. The International Committee of the Red Cross (ICRC) responds in situations of conflict and CHE. The activities of both the IFRC and ICRC also extend beyond disaster management.

Médecins Sans Frontières (MSF), another renowned humanitarian organization heavily involved in disaster relief, was founded in 1971 following war in Biafra. Its establishment was an important chapter in the history of the development, refinement and increasing professionalization of disaster relief work.

The WHO was formed in 1948 and has played an increasing role in the development and coordination of disaster response via the 2005 International Health Regulations Treaty (Burkle and Redmond, 2012) and its Inter-Agency Standing Committee's Health Cluster lead agencies.

More recently, disaster medicine has emerged as a medical specialty, heavily embedded in a multidisciplinary context. The next section of this chapter explores work and training opportunities within this area.

FOREIGN MEDICAL TEAMS (FMTS) AND INTERNATIONAL MEDICAL AID

International assistance is required when local capacity is exceeded. This might be to meet direct needs resulting from the disaster or to provide routine healthcare. For many FMTs the provision of surgical and trauma care is core business when augmenting the response to sudden onset disasters. These teams are one aspect of the broader disaster health response.

FMTS AND EBOLA

In August 2014, the WHO declared the Ebola outbreak in West Africa an international public health emergency. As it emerged, some organizations were already working in the hardest-hit countries of Guinea, Liberia and Sierra Leone (see Chapter 3).

Ebola demonstrated the complex interaction of poverty, inadequate health systems, politics and disease outbreak. In a highly developed nation (such as the UK) with mature and effective systems of acute healthcare, a single case of Ebola would not have the same potential to initiate disaster that it has had in areas of post-war dysfunction and extreme poverty, such as Sierra Leone.

The anticipated need for foreign medical professionals for the Ebola outbreak warrants consideration. The scale of the disaster meant that FMTs were required, but not surgical and anaesthetic units. Ebola required general medical professionals with an understanding of public health and tropical medicine, the versatility to work in complicated circumstances and the experience to function under pressure.

Activity 15.4

It's easy to see the outbreak of Ebola in Sierra Leone, Guinea and Liberia as a disaster, whereas isolated cases of the same disease in the USA, Spain and other developed communities did not represent a disaster.

What about Nigeria? Was the 2014 Ebola outbreak in Nigeria a disaster? What factors led to the successful containment of Ebola in Nigeria in October 2014? Consider risks, such as overpopulated slums, and protective factors, such as preparedness and early response.

PROFESSIONALISM AND STANDARDS

The international response to the earthquake in Haiti on 12 January 2010 accelerated discussion of well-known challenges in coordinating the delivery of aid. Some improvements have been made in the area of effective, accountable, collaborative aid management, yet concerns remain.

The Steering Committee for Humanitarian Response is an alliance of leading humanitarian organizations aiming to improve the services delivered to people in times of crisis. It has identified such problems as, 'people affected by crises do not consistently receive relevant and effective support from organizations claiming to assist them; nor do organizations consistently hold themselves accountable to them' (Tamminga, 2014: 1). Increasing professionalization and adherence to professional standards in disaster health is necessary. Non-maleficence must precede and augment beneficence.

The WHO's FMT Working Group cites concerns with coordination of the international medical response. Its publication (Norton et al., 2013) deals with FMTs providing trauma and surgical care. FMTs are expected to register in the country of response, declare their capacity and adhere to the principles and minimum standards for the category to which they belong. This is an important step forward in regulating international medical respondents. Countries in need of assistance select FMTs from the available registry and provide authorization for the team to work in their country. Applying FMT standards may, in turn, assist local health systems to develop their own standards and procedures. The WHO's publication strongly supports GEC systems, acknowledging, 'that the most timely and cost-effective response to trauma is the one mobilized by the affected country itself' and, 'the international community should support this approach for countries that do not have such capacity' (Norton et al., 2013: 20). Harmonization of specialized organizations towards improvement of local GEC capacity through the work of FMTs during a disaster health response can improve professional and ethical accountability.

DEVELOPING SKILLS AND EXPERIENCE IN GEC

A unique set of skills, knowledge and attributes is required for safe and effective GEC practice. Although it is not essential to travel abroad to engage in GEC activities, most globally minded EC clinicians undertake some form of fieldwork. This section provides practical advice on preparing to deliver and develop EC in low-resource environments.

ETHICAL CONSIDERATIONS

Although clinicians generally have a positive impact on the communities they serve, overseas placements can have unintended consequences. Successful assignments ensure mutual and reciprocal benefits for both the visiting health professionals and the host institutions. Chapter 1 introduced the ethical challenges for students and health professionals of working in developing settings. Observance of ethical principles is especially important in GEC activities because host populations are often vulnerable. Prior to departure, health professionals should ensure their assignment plan adheres to ethical guidelines. An important message for junior professionals is that, in disaster situations, professional and ethical responsibilities require practitioners to be appropriately trained and skilled for the tasks that will need to be undertaken.

SKILL AREAS AND TRAINING OPPORTUNITIES

EC professionals possess many qualities that are critical in GEC, including generalist medical knowledge and the capacity to function in volatile and stressful environments. Working in LMICs, however, requires a broader set of technical and non-technical skills that may not be acquired in the course of the conventional education of health professionals. All global health practitioners require basic skills in public health, communication, project management and cross-cultural engagement (Akbar et al., 2005). Attributes such as flexibility, resilience and self-awareness are also desirable.

Beyond these foundation competencies, clinicians active in GEC require expertise in the development and implementation of EC systems that can be adapted to local contexts. Dedicated GEC training programmes exist, predominantly in the USA, in the form of international EM (IEM) fellowships. These tend to be undertaken by emergency physicians after specialty training (www.iemfellowships.com/programs.php). Reviews of IEM fellowship curricula report several core elements (including tropical medicine, disaster health, humanitarian assistance, academia, project management and public health) and the following paragraphs provide practical suggestions as to how to build skills and knowledge in many of these areas (Bayram et al., 2010; Sistenich, 2012). Individuals should develop a learning strategy relevant to their work plans.

CLINICAL SKILLS AND EXPERTISE, INCLUDING TRAVEL, FIELD AND TROPICAL MEDICINE

All clinicians involved with medical aid and development activities must have the appropriate clinical capacity to do so, but the specific skill set required will depend on an individual's particular role. Although there are many relevant textbooks and online resources, the African Federation for Emergency Medicine's (AFEM) *AFEM Handbook of Acute and Emergency Care* (2014; see also the AFEM's website at: www.afem.info/resources/afem-handbook/?id=48) provides a comprehensive overview of the clinical skills and knowledge relevant to practising in LMICs. MSF's *Clinical Guidelines* manual (2013) is another useful resource and is available online.

Prior to deploying abroad, clinicians should develop a broad base of skills by training in a number of different disciplines and environments. Working locally with underserviced populations (for instance, migrant groups and indigenous communities) is likely to provide valuable experience.

Skills in tropical and travel medicine can be obtained through short courses and degree programmes. Prominent examples include the diploma courses offered by the Liverpool School of Tropical Medicine and the London School of Hygiene and Tropical Medicine (both in the UK), as well as the Gorgas Course in Clinical Tropical Medicine, taught in English in Peru. Other institutions offering programmes include Johns Hopkins University (USA), James Cook University (Australia) and the Bangkok School of Tropical Medicine (Thailand).

DISASTER HEALTH

At a national level, governments and NGOs often facilitate training in responding to disasters and provide ongoing coordination and support for deployable medical assistance teams. In the UK, the Department of International Development relies on the charity UK-Med to train its health professionals and facilitate deployments.

Other options for developing skills include:

- locally organized disaster response simulation exercises, such as the desktop Emergo Train System
- meetings of the World Association for Disaster and Emergency Management
- the ICRC's Health Emergencies in Large Populations (HELP) course
- NGO and university courses, such as those listed on the website of the UK's Enhancing Learning and Research for Humanitarian Assistance (ELRHA: www.elrha.org) – simply enter 'courses' in the 'Search' window).

TRAINING OPPORTUNITIES THROUGH NETWORKS, ORGANIZATIONS AND ACADEMIC INSTITUTIONS

Knowledge and contacts can be developed through engagement with established GEC networks. Internationally, IFEM has a key role in promoting EM specialty development. In Africa, AFEM is the peak body for EC and has played a pivotal role in increasing its profile. A number of HICs also have dedicated IEM networks through their peak bodies, such as the Australasian College for Emergency Medicine and the American College of Emergency Physicians.

Several academic, government and non-governmental organizations are involved in GEC activities, providing opportunities for health professionals early in their careers to further develop their skills and gain field experience. For those clinicians enrolled in an EM training programme, supervised overseas deployments may be recognized towards training requirements.

Relatively few university departments dedicated to GEC exist. In the USA, several institutions offer opportunities in research as well as fieldwork, such as the Harvard Humanitarian Initiative and the Johns Hopkins Centre for Refugee and Disaster Response.

Many hospitals, universities and EM societies have relationships with over-seas institutions. These types of partnerships may involve long-term placements, large-scale workforce development programmes and/or discrete training courses. Such partnerships are often long-term ones, with development projects and out-comes outlasting individual participants' involvement. They are commonly reciprocal in nature, too, allowing staff from LMICs to experience EC in developed settings.

Volunteering is a common way for health professionals early in their careers to gain experience in global health. Organizations include:

- Peace Corps (USA)
- Voluntary Service Overseas (VSO) International
- Australian Volunteers International.

In crisis situations and CHEs, NGOs usually provide the bulk of medical assistance. Organizations with particular expertise in EC include MSF, the ICRC and International Rescue Committee. A small number of NGOs focus exclusively on developing the capacity for EC in low-resource settings. One example is shown in the following case study of the Global Emergency Care Collaborative.

Case study   Global Emergency Care Collaborative

The mission of the Global Emergency Care Collaborative (GECC) is to improve global health by enhancing access to quality EC in the developing world by collaborating with local and national organizations. The shortage of acute care services in sub-Saharan Africa results in a large burden of preventable morbidity and mortality, precluding the region from achieving the health-related MDGs. The majority of children who die in sub-Saharan African hospitals do so within 24 hours of arrival.

The GECC, an NGO founded by emergency physicians in the USA, addresses these problems by developing a sustainable horizontal acute care system and training providers from multiple health cadres in acute care delivery for the full continuum of illness and injury. By performing assessments of community needs, working alongside medical practitioners and directly caring for patients, the GECC is improving access to EC by training local providers and introducing appropriate medical technology.

The role of the WHO in GEC is generally limited to public health emergencies and humanitarian crises, where it has a coordinating function through its Health Cluster. Other UN agencies, such as the Office for the Coordination of Humanitarian

Affairs (OCHA), occasionally require expertise in GEC. Opportunities for clinicians in these organizations are limited, although internships are available.

Military medical units are often involved in trauma management in the context of war and civil unrest, but this aspect of EC is beyond the traditional definition of global health. Defence forces tend to become involved with humanitarian crises when the local civilian organizations are overrun.

CHALLENGES AND PROSPECTS FOR CAREER DEVELOPMENT

Barriers to engaging in GEC activities include competing demands of clinical training, examinations, research, financial constraints and domestic commitments. The experiences of EM trainees who have worked extensively in LMICs illustrate the benefits as well as the challenges of undertaking GEC activities early in one's career (Thurtle et al., 2014).

CONCLUSION

This chapter has provided an overview of GEC and disaster health. EC has a central role in health systems and, due to disaster situations, complex and humanitarian emergencies and daily health needs, the global requirement for safe and effective acute care is increasing. So, too, therefore, is the need for highly skilled GEC practitioners.

Organizations with useful websites for further information include the IFEM (www.ifem.cc), IFRC (www.ifrc.org), MSF (www.msf.org.uk), the UN's Sustainable Development Knowledge Platform (https://sustainabledevelopment.un.org) and the WHO's FMT Working Group (www.who.int/hac/global_health_cluster/fmt/en).

REFERENCES

AFEM (2014) *AFEM Handbook of Acute and Emergency Care*. Oxford: Cape Town: University Press Southern Africa.

Akbar, H., Hill, P., Rotem, A., Riley, I., Zwi, A. and Marks, G. (2005) 'Identifying competencies for Australian health professionals working in international health', *Asia Pacific Journal of Public Health*, 17(2): 99–103.

Bayram, J., Rosborough, S., Bartels, S., Lis, J., VanRooyen, M.J., Kapur, B. and Anderson, P.D. (2010) 'Core curricular elements for fellowship training in international emergency medicine', *Academic Emergency Medicine*, 17(7): 748–757.

Becker, T., Jacquet, G., Marsh, R., Schroeder, E., Foran, M., Bartels, S., et al. (2014) 'Global emergency medicine: a review of the literature from 2013', *Academic Emergency Medicine*, 21(7): 810–817.

Burkle, F. and Redmond, A. (2012) 'An authority for crisis coordination and accountability', *The Lancet*, 379: 2223–2225.

Curry, C. (2008) 'A perspective on developing emergency medicine as a specialty', *International Journal of Emergency Medicine*, 1(3): 163–167.

Médecins San Frontières (MSF) (2013) *Clinical Guidelines: Diagnosis and Treatment Manual*. Paris: Médecins San Frontières. Available online at: www.refbooks.msf.org (accessed 8 October 2015).

Molyneux, E., Ahmad, S. and Robertson, A. (2006) 'Improved triage and emergency care for children reduces inpatient mortality in a resource constrained setting', *Bulletin of the World Health Organization*, 84: 314–319.

Norton, I., von Schreeb, J., Aitken, P., Herard, P. and Lajolo, C. (2013) *Classification and Minimum Standards for Foreign Medical Teams in Sudden Onset Disasters*. Global Health Cluster. Geneva, World Health Organization.

Phillips, G.A., Soe, Z.W., Kong, J.H.B. and Curry, C. (2014) 'Capacity Building for Emergency Care: Training the First Emergency Specialists in Myanmar', *Emergency Medicine Australasia*, 26(6): 618–26.

Razzak, J.A. and Kellermann, A.L. (2002) 'Emergency medical care in developing countries: is it worthwhile?', *Bulletin of the World Health Organization*, 80(10): 900–905.

Redmond, A.D. (2005) 'ABC of conflict and disaster: natural disasters', *British Medical Journal*, 330: 1259–1261.

Sistenich, V. (2012) 'International emergency medicine: how to train for it', *Emergency Medicine Australasia*, 24(4): 435–441.

Tamminga, P. (2014) *Certification Review Project: Summary of Key Findings and Recommendations*. Steering Committee for Humanitarian Response.

Thurtle, N., Phillips, G., Keage, J., Wallis, A., Mitchell, R. and Jamieson, J. (2014) 'Perspectives on working and training in global health and international emergency medicine', *Emergency Medicine Australasia*, 26: 635–639.

United Nations Development Programme Bureau for Crisis Prevention and Recovery (2004) *Reducing Disaster Risk: A Challenge for Development*. New York: United Nations.

World Health Organization (2005) *Emergency Triage Assessment and Treatment: Manual for Participants*. Geneva: WHO.

16

PROJECT PLANNING AND EVALUATION

ANN K. ALLEN

Chapter overview

After reading this chapter you will be able to:

- explain the contribution projects can make to improving global health
- identify health priorities
- identify and engage with relevant stakeholders
- select an intervention
- secure funding
- describe what a manager does
- use three 'rules' to help you manage others
- monitor and evaluate.

INTRODUCTION

Healthcare provision involves, 'complex, amorphous mobilisations of human activities and resources that vary significantly from one locale to another, embedded in and influenced by complex political and social networks' (Herman et al., 1987: 9) Consequently, it is important to not only take account of the specific epidemiological patterns of disease in the setting in which you are to work but also be sensitive to the population that is to be served – its demographic composition, cultural practices and values and the distribution of power, as well as the socio-economic resources at its disposal.

The use of projects to provide health services enables management, 'to accomplish unique outcomes with limited resources under critical time constraints' (Meredith and Mantel, 1989: v). The use of projects enables an organization to plan, organize, implement and control its activities and how it uses its staff and resources. This chapter addresses how this works in practice.

PROJECTS AND PROGRAMMES

A 'project' is any activity that brings together people, resources and activities directed towards the achievement of a specified goal within a defined timeframe. A project may be small, such as planning and running a series of advocacy workshops over a few months to raise awareness of the needs of people with disabilities in order to get a government policy to promote 'disability rights'. It may have more diverse objectives with a timeframe measured in years. An example of this might be the development of hospital- and community-based palliative care provision, as happened in Kenya with support from the British Joint Funding Scheme (JFS) over several years in the 1990s. The JFS later became known as the Civil Society Unit. The objectives here were to raise funds to provide facilities, train teams of staff and raise awareness about palliative care in members of the public and professionals alike.

'Programmes' are projects containing a very large number of interventions, such as UNICEF's multi-country Accelerated Child Survival and Development programme, implemented in eleven countries in West Africa from 2001 until 2005. It introduced 14 interventions (Bryce et al., 2010).

Projects are often used to 'test the water' before embedding provision into mainstream health services. Sometimes they are the only way in which some provision to meet local health needs can be made. NGOs can solicit funding from donor agencies and private corporations to run projects that the country's government cannot afford to provide. Activity 16.1 encourages you to find out how an affiliate of Johns Hopkins University, Jhpiego, is currently saving lives.

--------------------------------- Activity 16.1 ---------------------------------

Watch the YouTube video 'Jhpiego – the Force of 40 Years' (at: www.youtube.com/watch?v=8cXCMYzdZhE&feature=youtu.be). It is 6.48 minutes long.

What is Jhpiego's mission? Note down the names of the different organizations with which it has partnered, either by receiving technical support or financial donations.

Comment

By taking the scientific knowledge developed in resource-rich countries and training local staff in their own country to implement evidence-based practice, health practitioners can serve their communities more effectively than if they were to study in the USA. For instance, in Ghana, a public–private partnership of the Ghana Health Service, Jhpiego and the Jubilee Partners formed the STAR CHPS project to build the capacity of health service providers to engage with communities to improve their health in 61 facilities across six coastal districts of Ghana.

As we saw in Chapter 3, one way to address people's health needs is to use scarce, trained health professionals to provide training, supervision and support to communities, thereby freeing experts' time so they can provide more of the more complex clinical care needed. This extends the reach of healthcare provision efficiently.

What is the evidence?

As a community health nurse (CHN) running a small clinic in Ellembelle District, Ghana, Joseph Opoku Cobbinah knew how to deliver basic healthcare to the people who came to the Aidoo Suazo Community-based Health Planning and Services (CHPS) compound. His clients, however, were few and far from the clinic and Cobbinah did not know how to change that.

Then, thanks to the Jubilee Partners' Supportive Technical Assistance for Revitalizing Community-based Health Planning and Services (STAR CHPS) project, Cobbinah received the training and support he needed to connect with community leaders and health volunteers, reach more people in his district and provide quality services. In a series of activities led by Jhpiego, Cobbinah learned new skills in various areas, including reproductive and child health, family planning, communicating beneficial changes to behaviour, mobilization of the community, prevention of infection, HIV/AIDS and emergency deliveries.

'Now that I had both the knowledge and skills to work with the community, I was able to more effectively engage them in my work,' Cobbinah said. 'I had a directional sign for the facility constructed to ensure that community members knew where I was located. I spent time educating community members about important health topics, such as malaria. I encouraged and supported community health volunteers to bring community members to see me. As a result of these combined efforts, the number of people benefiting from services has increased.' So satisfied was the local community that they bought him a motorbike so that he could reach even more people (Jhpiego, 2013).

A follow-up evaluation of Cobbinah's activities, showing his success in making improvements, means that he is now training other CHNs for the project. This kind of cascading is typical for many project activities in health.

The following sections outline the stages of project development.

IDENTIFYING HEALTH PRIORITIES

Often you will be employed on a project where these decisions have already been made, but it is useful to know about the different ways in which health priorities can be identified. Changes are often sparked by some sort of crisis arising within the organization or external events. A sudden rise in the incidence of a hospital-acquired infection (HAI), such as meticillin-resistant *Staphylococcus aureus* (MRSA), for example, would generate a project to minimize the risks of future outbreaks. See the following case study for an example of such a situation.

Case study   Identification of a health problem

Consistent hand washing or the use of alcohol-based gel (except for *C. difficile*) is a necessity in preventing transmission from colonized or infected patients to other patients on the hands of healthcare workers. Screening or surveillance cultures for MRSA or vancomyscin-resistant *Enterococcus* (VRE) are performed at many hospitals on admission in an early effort to identify colonized patients who may then serve as a source of infection. Any patient identified as having *C. difficile*, MRSA or VRE colonization or infection is then placed on contact isolation precautions (this requires the use of a gown and gloves). Strict cleaning of the environment is then needed any time there is turnover within the hospital room.

While these screening and isolation measures have shown decreasing rates of HAI in studies across the UK, most studies do not separate the interventions, making it difficult to determine which ones are the most effective (Kelly and Monson, 2012: 644)

A project might also be undertaken in order to raise the profile of an issue to influence policy and make it a priority concern, as when Mayon-White et al. (1988), on the recommendations of a WHO advisory group convened for this purpose, measured the prevalence of HAI in 47 hospitals. This international study (14 countries across Europe, Asia, Australia and the Middle East) used a standardized protocol to survey patients. Its results informed a programme for the control and prevention of HAI.

A recent two-year project for the prevention of cervical cancer in Burkina Faso by the NGO Jhpiego increased government awareness of the situation and strengthened political commitment to developing a national, comprehensive cervical cancer prevention strategy that uses a 'single visit approach, ... [with] visual inspection of the cervix after applying acetic acid (vinegar) to the cervix and, if indicated, treatment of precancerous lesions by cryotherapy during the same visit. Providing all of these services in one visit reduces the proportion of women lost to follow-up' (Jhpiego, 2012: 2).

Activity 16.2

Why might follow-up be a problem? Make a few notes of your ideas.

Comment

Burkina Faso is an extremely poor country, with a very low rate of literacy and a high dependence on subsistence agriculture. A woman who has attended a clinic, perhaps for antenatal care, is unlikely to recognize the seriousness of a condition that a doctor (or nurse) has identified as a precancerous lesion. She may not feel her need for treatment is worth the monetary and time costs of returning to the clinic when she has both farming and domestic duties to attend to – in other words, her opportunity costs exceed the perceived benefits.

An assessment of need by measuring the incidence and prevalence of a health problem or a disease identifies the potential benefits. Need differs from demand, which is what people might wish to use (where healthcare is free at the point of delivery) or what they would be willing to pay for if not. The Burkina Faso example illustrates why there may be no demand for a perceived need. Supply is what is actually provided and, under these specific local conditions, the proposed single visit approach will help to reduce the prevalence of cervical cancer.

In poor countries such as Burkina Faso, decisions will be made on the basis of epidemiologically determined need when cost-effective solutions exist – the selective approach to PHC adopted by UNICEF in the 1980s. Health needs assessments may also take account of the distribution of the needs by comparing different localities with similar demographic structures (Cavanagh and Chadwick, 2009). They can be used to justify incremental changes to existing services, rectify health inequalities and manage supply and demand where different stakeholders (politicians, professionals and the public) hold different views.

IDENTIFY AND ENGAGE WITH RELEVANT STAKEHOLDERS

Stakeholders are those (groups of) people who have either a direct or an indirect interest in your project and, thus, in the results of any evaluation. They may also be in a position to obstruct or promote the implementation of your project. So, you need to think about how each audience might draw a benefit from (have a stake in) or be disadvantaged by a change in the status quo if the intervention is effective.

Stakeholders' involvement and sense of ownership are critical elements for a successful project. Communication and collaborative working are the means for securing this engagement. Remember that communication involves dialogue, which, in turn, means listening to other points of view. Failure to do this results in inefficiencies or worse. For instance, it does not make sense to decide unilaterally on the processes and outcomes to be recorded in information systems on which future evaluations will be based. Stakeholders will value different outputs, so, while all may agree that a reduced prevalence of the disease is desired, some will be concerned also about the impact on the quality and safety of healthcare, with changes in workload or recognition or the implications for their performance of the service. A decision by medical staff to change the format of reporting of genetic disorders (to make it easier for them to assimilate the information) may have consequences for the laboratory service providers, who appreciate better than the clinicians how current reporting is tied in to particular software systems and how even minor change necessitates shutting down the current system in order to test the new one (with implications for providing ongoing diagnostic services).

SELECTING AN INTERVENTION

Healthcare includes not only treatment but also prevention, diagnosis (and the reassurance it can bring), continuing care for long-term conditions, rehabilitation and palliative care. What is selected will reflect the cost-effectiveness of the intervention as well as its acceptability (to professionals and the public – in particular, the patients) and the feasibility of its being delivered safely. In some areas where schistosomiasis is endemic, for example, it may be more cost-effective to treat people with the disease with Praziquantel (which is an effective, non-toxic and inexpensive drug) than seek to prevent its transmission by killing snails, particularly as reducing the number of people shedding eggs could itself impact transmission. Equally, genital infection with *Schistosoma haemotobium* has been shown in a cross-sectional study in Zimbabwe to be associated with a three-fold risk of having HIV-1 (Kjetland et al., 2006), which has led to discussion about the potential for widening the scope of treatment for the drug. Comparisons based on cost-effectiveness are sensitive to what is included in the measurement: vaccination programmes are highly cost-effective in terms of YLLs as they benefit young children, but it does mean that the needs of elderly people at greater risk of heart disease and cancers have lower priority afforded to them.

The Nairobi Terminal Care project referred to earlier arose from a review by Kenyan health professionals that concluded a charitable organization should be established to provide care and support for the terminally ill and their families. The late Professor Edward George Kasili chaired a board of trustees that led to the registration of a charitable trust and fundraising to build a one-storey centre close to Kenyatta Hospital. This was officially opened in 1990 and was the seed that grew into the Kenya Hospices and Palliative Care Association (KEHPCA), although, as yet, palliative care provision has not been embedded into the Kenyan health service. Training of community-based volunteers, nurses and doctors followed, based on an exchange scheme with the Trent Region Palliative and Continuing Care Centre (TRPCCC). This enabled Kenyan staff to build their expertise in the UK, while experienced UK staff provided support to set up an effective domiciliary service and contributed to teaching in Nairobi. It was intended by the TRPCCC that training would be multidisciplinary, with teams working together and training together, but each cadre received separate training.

Although Professor Kasili saw no difficulty in having a nurse in authority over a doctor when the senior nursing officer was appointed to be the project coordinator, he also explained his objection to holding combined courses for doctors and nurses by stating that doctors felt threatened by nurses, who had more experience in patient care. Doctors at Nairobi's private hospital were reluctant to refer patients to the hospice because it meant a loss of income and involvement in private practice in the evenings affected their attendance at training courses. Most palliative care units in the country today are headed or run by a nurse and KEHPCA is advocating the development of a policy to allow nurses to prescribe opioids, for which they are not currently certified.

Another factor in selecting an intervention will be the availability of funding, which, in turn, reflects current donor's interests. The WHO's increased concern to address the rise of NCDs may be prompted partly by the social consequences of people being too poor to pay for medical care, whether in New York, Australia or Madurai, India. While there are NGOs and charities that may offer support, care of the elderly is not high on any government's agenda, nor those of multilateral organizations.

Case study

Cases of elderly people being abandoned by poor families is on the rise.

In Madurai, India, in the twilight of their lives, elderly people have been abandoned in hospital by relatives who are either unable to care for them or don't want to shoulder responsibility.

Octogenarian S. Vellaimmal, a resident of Manchanaickanpatti on the outskirts of Madurai, can barely remember anything. Her daughter is alive, but has left her at the government-owned Rajaji Hospital, say the staff. The case of M. Vasantha (75) of Madurai is similar. So is that of Damodharan (60) of Valliyur, who is bedridden and has lost his vision and speech. They were all in hospital for a month and, after their relatives could not be traced, were shifted to an old age home (Sivaraman, 2011).

Project planning requires you to be able to identify sources of funding and actively engage with potential donors. The following activity will prepare you for doing this.

—————————————— Activity 16.3 ——————————————

Search on the Internet to find an example of a project to support elders abandoned by their families at a religious festival, at home or in a hospital that is looking for funding.

Comment

You may have found something different from some of the results of my search below – so much the better for opportunities for elder well-being!

Maitri India is constructing an Ageing Resource Centre in Vrindavan, which will be a home to 100 elderly and destitute widow mothers. The centre will also offer facilities for empowering them through vocational training and employment opportunities. It is soliciting donations through 'Global Giving' (www.globalgiving.org) to purchase furniture and equipment to create a safe and comfortable home.

In the UK, the Almshouse Association is launching a sixty-fifth anniversary appeal to extend its fund for member almshouse charities (www.almshouses.org). Age UK (www.ageuk.org.uk) and Age International (www.ageinternational.org.uk) raise funds to support elderly people and advocate on their behalf.

While the Bill & Melinda Gates Foundation has a funding stream for pneumonia, it states, 'While pneumonia affects people of all ages, our priority is children under age 5.'

SECURING FUNDING

An advantage of asking local industries and entrepreneurs for help is that funding is more likely to be sustained and offerings 'in kind' may also be available – as with the Kenyan Ministry of Health, which provided land for the hospice building, although it could not offer cash.

If you are approaching NGOs, it is important to pay close attention to what they will *not* fund. For instance, the Bill & Melinda Gates Foundation does not support applications for:

- direct donations or grants to individuals
- projects addressing health problems in developed countries

- political campaigns and legislative lobbying efforts
- building or capital campaigns
- projects that exclusively serve religious purposes.

You also need to note what information is required in an application and make sure you comply with any instructions, including deadlines. Make sure you demonstrate how your proposal fits with the donor's requirements in a covering letter (and in the proposal itself). Although this letter is written last, prepare it carefully. It should be neatly laid out, with no spelling mistakes, for instance. A bad impression will be difficult to make up for later. It determines how well the rest of the proposal is received. You'll want to address your letter to a specific person, briefly state what your proposal is asking for and summarize the essence of your project.

Formats for proposals are fairly standard, whether you are applying to a foundation or a government. Succinctness, relevance and clarity are important throughout. The format to follow is this.

1. Executive summary

This summary comes after your cover letter. It helps the funder to understand quickly what you are seeking. It can be as short as a couple of sentences, but not any longer than a page. Briefly touch on the main points of your proposal. You want to entice the reader to keep going. The summary should be well written (to impress), complete (explain what your organization does and its mission) and specific enough to show it meets the donor's objectives.

2. Needs assessment

Your aim is to convince the funder that what you propose to do is important and your organization is the right one to do it. Explain why the issue is important and what research you did to learn about possible solutions. You may have used analytical tools, such as problem and objective trees, SWOT and stakeholder analyses (Schmeer, 1999), and a risk matrix. SWOT stands for an organization's strengths, weaknesses, opportunities and threats, which need to be described, compared and evaluated.

Do include both stories and data, and match these to the interests of the funder. Show how this project solves an important societal problem and why the funder should be interested in supporting it.

3. Aims and objectives (also referred to as impacts and outcomes) and targets

Here is where you explain what your project plans to do about the problem. State what you ultimately hope to accomplish with the project and spell out the specific results or outcomes you expect to accomplish. Think of aims as very general, broad outcomes (for example, to improve women's health) and objectives as the outcomes or what will have changed if your project is successful (to reduce maternal mortality). Targets are the specific steps you'll take to get to those outcomes (increase the uptake of antenatal care or improve the uptake of tetanus vaccination), making sure these targets are SMART (specific, measurable, attainable, relevant and time-bound).

4. **Implementation of the project**

This is where you explain to the funder exactly how you will achieve the goals and objectives you set out earlier. You may be required to use a logical framework in this section (DFID, 2011). If you do, then there is a place to explain how you will monitor and evaluate progress, including the indicators for success that you will use. Make this section very detailed and logical. Include a timeline and specify who will do what and by when. In planning your project, it makes sense to start agreeing what you want to achieve (impacts/outcomes), then identify the outputs, activities and inputs needed to achieve them. It's an iterative process, but using a log frame enables you to keep the plan alive to respond to changing circumstances.

5. **Evaluation of the project**

Funders want to know that their contributions actually did some good. So, decide from the start how you will evaluate your project's impact. State what records you will keep or data you will collect and how you will use that data. Include the costs of data collection in your budget. Employing a credible person outside of your organization to do this ensures that an evaluation is seen to be objective.

6. **Budget, funding and sustainability**

Ensure that the budget is complete, realistic and carefully laid out. Most funders do not wish to be the sole source of support for a project, so be sure to mention in-kind contributions you expect, such as meeting space or equipment, as well as any other expected sources of funding. Is this a pilot project with a limited timeline or will it continue? If so, how do you plan to fund it? Is it sustainable? Some donors also like to know about compliance with policies, such as gender equality.

7. **Organizational information**

Briefly explain what your organization does and why the funder can trust it to use the requested funds responsibly and effectively. Give a short history of your organization, state its mission, the population it serves and provide an overview of its track record in achieving its mission. Describe or list previous or current projects. Even if you know the funder or have received funding from this source before, it's important to include this in your proposal.

WHAT DOES A MANAGER DO?

Like medicine and the health sciences, management is as much an art as it is a science. Some matters can be examined empirically in order to make predictions (such as examining epidemiological data regarding health needs in order to plan to meet future demands). Much more of a manager's time is spent on enabling individuals and groups of people (who sometimes are teams) to work together to meet the organization's goals. Managers integrate the activities of others so that the complex requirements of a health service can be met. They ensure that the resources, staff with the right skills and the environment (whether physical, social or psychological) are co-present so that a team can function effectively. They may need to intervene in breakdowns of communication or where there are conflicts of interest. Sometimes they intervene to resolve outright conflict that not only prevents the accomplishment of tasks but also puts the well-being of ancillary staff at risk. On a more positive note, their ability to recognize good work and excellent performance can promote morale and ensure staff are given recognition and opportunities to progress.

Activity 16.4

Identifying a manager's role

You can use a part-time job, a clinical placement or even casual observation to answer the following question. What do you think managers do? You may have heard people say that managers are unnecessary – can you think of reasons to agree with this? How might you refute the points you make?

Comment

I wonder how far your list of what managers do agrees with that of Mintzberg (1989)? Mintzberg's research in HICs led him to identify the real behaviour of managers (not all of whom were hospital administrators by a long chalk). He identified ten 'roles':

- figurehead, leader and liaison are interpersonal roles
- informational roles comprise acting as a monitor, spokesperson and disseminator
- decisionmaking aspects of the position involve being an entrepreneur, a disturbance handler, resource allocator and a negotiator.

Effective managers learn to resist daily job pressures and use analytical tools in order to form an overview of current circumstances. You may feel that, as responsible professionals concerned to promote others' well-being, you do not need to be managed. Mintzberg concluded, however, that managers are needed to ensure the efficiency and effectiveness of activities, and meet their organization's purposes (and those of their clients). Managers clarify organizational aims and objectives to staff and ensure that structures are suitably designed to facilitate the meeting of those objectives. They act as an informational intermediary between the organization and the outside world, while, at the same time, developing strategies to ensure the organization can adapt to this wider environment. It is necessary to hold formal authority so as to be able to negotiate credibly and manage staff disputes.

In the public sector, managers are constrained by policies set out with the organization they represent and, in LICs, cultural differences may also affect a manager's behaviour. The welfare of staff, for instance, may extend beyond health and safety at work to include contributing to their familial and personal well-being and even that of former members of staff.

MANAGING OTHERS

Iles (1997) proposes three 'rules' for managing people successfully. The first is to ensure that you agree exactly what it is you expect them to do. The second is that you and they are confident that they have the skills and resources they need to be successful. Last, but not least, give feedback on how well they are doing.

Managing expectations is best done face to face, with opportunities given to clarify exactly what is wanted. Remember, people come with expectations and assumptions based on previous experiences. If something is important to you, then spell it out. If you know that the report you are asking someone to write is just a starting point for negotiation with a budget controller, then you probably want current numbers which are 'good enough', neatly and succinctly presented with dates and sources; you are not expecting in-depth research of difficult-to-access information, so be clear about the boundaries. Support them in finding relevant information by telling them where to search and check progress regularly so they don't go down a blind alley.

Activity 16.5

This activity is about trying out the three 'rules'.

Think about someone you think could benefit from some feedback from you. It might be someone in your team or a classmate and the feedback could be about something he or she is currently doing or has done or else it might be something he or she is not doing. Prepare what you will say, where and how, using Iles' (1997) guidelines. Then ask a friend how well you are observing the guidelines. Notice how you feel about the feedback you receive.

Comment

Feedback involves a dialogue and it should be constructive. This can be difficult if the person resents being given advice or feels threatened by being managed by someone whom they believe to be unsuitable.

Managers, while being respectful of others, should not be seeking popularity but be concerned with achieving the organization's goals by making the best use of the people they are responsible for. This takes emotional intelligence and hard work.

MONITORING AND EVALUATION

The life cycle of every project includes regular monitoring of activities and processes, together with evaluation of outcomes and impacts. This encourages ownership and participation through working closely with project partners and other stakeholders. It also ensures resources are used effectively and efficiently to deliver outputs/ outcomes within the agreed budget. By recording evidence of what is and is not working, important lessons are learned for design and implementation of future projects.

Performance success is judged through using relevant indicators of progress against specified targets. They should be specific, useable and measurable. Each indicator you choose to measure your objectives must be verifiable by some means – through administrative records or even a survey initiated specifically for that purpose. If not, you must find another indicator. Obviously it is cheapest to make good use of routinely collected data.

Outcomes should identify what will change and who will benefit from the project. They may show how the project will contribute to reducing poverty or to the MDGs or whatever the stakeholders have agreed as a priority. It should be clear how an outcome contributes to the higher-level situation or its impact in collaboration with other projects.

Outputs are the specific, direct deliverables of the project, such as a report, data analysis or intervention. These will provide the conditions necessary to achieve the outcomes. The logic of the chain from outputs to outcomes therefore needs to be clear. Milestones for the objectives should be set at appropriate intervals.

The individual characteristics of your project will show what monitoring data should be reviewed and summarized weekly, monthly or quarterly. Reviews are intended to help you track progress. Planning this helps with the sequencing of activities, as well as the release of data from the source of the monitoring information and allows you to check that the right resources will be available when needed because budgets are tied to the activities required in the outputs. Project management (PM) software or planning tools, such as Gantt charts, help plan and track progress against goals and timelines.

Evaluation of progress, while used for reasons of accountability, should also be to learn from the process. If something is not working, it's important to try and understand why.

Dissemination is the final stage of the project. Depending on how or whether the project was funded, this might take the form of a report to a funding body or key stakeholders, a presentation to stakeholders or at a conference, an article in a peer-reviewed journal or information posted on a website. Dissemination is important to share successes and failures, lessons learned and indicate next steps for research.

CONCLUSION

A project-based approach encourages the efficient use of scarce resources in a complex and dynamic world and the synergy promoted by collaborative working between organizations and with communities makes it possible to 'scale up' the impact of individual projects and learn lessons from other settings. The engagement of stakeholders through the development of planning and evaluation is important for the success and sustainability of a project. In planning a project, it is vital to know the context in which it will be implemented, make use of all the evidence that has been collected regarding what is needed and what works and to know where to go for funding (and, thus, take account of the potential donor's interests and values).

Managing people requires attentiveness from the manager. Recognize that it is inevitable people will bring different expectations and interests to the situation and practise Iles' three rules. His rules of monitoring, evaluation and dissemination address the need to be accountable, but can also provide valuable lessons about what is needed for a project to be a success and help others working on similar issues or problems.

REFERENCES

Bryce, J., Gilroy, K., Jones, G., Hazel, E., Black, R.E. and Victora, C.G. (2010) 'The Accelerated Child Survival and Development programme in West Africa: a retrospective evaluation', *The Lancet*, 375: 572–582.

Cavanagh, S. and Chadwick, K. (2009) *Health Needs Assessment: A Practical Guide*. London: NICE [ed.]NICE. p. 105. Available at: www.urbanreproductivehealth.org/toolkits/measuring-success/health-needs-assessment-practical-guide

DFID (2011) *Guidance on Using the Revised Logical Framework*. Available at: www.gov.uk/government/uploads/system/uploads/attachment_data/file/67638/how-to-guid-rev-log-fmwk.pdf (accessed 8 October 2015).

Herman, J.L., Morris, L.L. and Fitz-Gibbon, C.T. (1987) *Evaluators Handbook*. Newbury Park, CA: SAGE.

Iles, V. (1997) *Really Managing Healthcare*. Buckingham: Open University Press.

Jhpiego (2012) *Jhpiego in Burkina Faso*. Available at: www.jhpiego.org/files/Burkina%20 Faso%20Country%20Profile.pdf (accessed 8 October 2015).

Jhpiego (2013) *A STAR Shines: Jubilee Partners Project Develops Strong Community Health Leaders*. Available at: www.jhpiego.org/content/star-shines-jubilee-partners-project-develops-strong-community-health-leaders (accessed 8 October 2015).

Kelly, K.N. and Monson, J.R.T. (2012) 'Hospital-acquired infections', *Surgery (Oxford)*, 30: 640–644.

Kjetland, E., Ndhlovu, P.D., Gomo, E., Mduluza, T., Midzi, N., Gwanzura, L., Mason, P.R., et al. (2006) 'Association between genital schistosomiasis and HIV in rural Zimbabwean women', *AIDS*, 20: 593–600.

Mayon-White, R.T., Ducel, G., Kereselidze, T. and Tikomirov, E. (1988) 'An international survey of the prevalence of hospital-acquired infection', *Journal of Hospital Infection*, 11 (Supplement A): 43–48.

Meredith, J.R. and Mantel, S.J. (1989) *Project Management: A Managerial Approach*, 2nd edition. Singapore: John Wiley & Sons.

Mintzberg, H. (1989) *Mintzberg on Management: Inside Our Strange World of Organizations*. New York: Free Press.

Schmeer, K. (1999) *Guidelines for Conducting a Stakeholder Analysis*. Bethesda, MD: Partnerships for Health Reform, Abt Associates Inc. Available at: www.who.int/management/partnerships/overall/GuidelinesConductingStakeholderAnalysis.pdf (accessed 8 October 2015).

Sivaraman, R. (2011) 'Cases of elderly abandoned by poor families on the rise'. Available at: http://articles.timesofindia.indiatimes.com/2011-10-04/madurai/30242172_1_age-home-rajaji-hospital-madurai (accessed 8 October 2015).

INDEX

Note: Page numbers in *italics* indicate figures and tables.